Breaking Free

Help for survivors of child sexual abuse

Third edition

KAY TOON AND CAROLYN AINSCOUGH

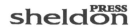

sheldon **PRESS**

First published in Great Britain in 1993

Sheldon Press
36 Causton Street
London SW1P 4ST
www.sheldonpress.co.uk

Second edition published 2000
Third edition published 2018

British Library Cataloguing-in-Publication Data
A catalogue record for this book is available from the British Library

ISBN 978–1–84709–465–0
eBook ISBN 978–1–84709–466–7

Typeset by Fakenham Prepress Solutions, Fakenham, Norfolk NR21 8NN
First printed in Great Britain by Ashford Colour Press
Subsequently digitally reprinted in Great Britain

eBook by Fakenham Prepress Solutions, Fakenham, Norfolk NR21 8NN

Produced on paper from sustainable forests

Contents

Foreword

Children exposed to sexual abuse give us a tragic insight into the untold damage such abuse generates. Often the consequences are devastating. The groundbreaking Adverse Childhood Experiences (ACEs) study (1998) highlighted how childhood experiences – both positive and negative – have the potential to shape the future probability of an individual becoming a victim or perpetrator of violence, lifelong physical and psychological health and well-being, and opportunities for the future. Early adverse childhood experiences represent the most pressing public health issue of our time. Child sexual abuse is a crime much greater than official statistics show – being often under-reported, undetected and insufficiently prosecuted.

In the early 1990s, I established two Adult Survivors of Childhood Sexual Abuse Networks – one on the Wirral (female survivors) and the other in Liverpool (male survivors). These networks were for adult mental health populations at a time when a psychiatric diagnosis was deemed separate from earlier experiences of child sexual abuse – although for some such a viewpoint pervades today. As a young mental health clinician, I came across Ainscough and Toon's *Breaking Free: Helping survivors of child sexual abuse* (1993). This book became an integral resource for me and was invaluable in best empowering me in working with survivors. It informed my practice enormously. What stood out for me were phenomenological patterns in survivors' journeys, discussed, for example, in the chapters on survival and recovery, speaking out, acknowledging the damage, wondering 'Why me?' and 'Why didn't I tell?', 'silent ways of telling' and so on. This book shaped my clinical practice, clinical supervision, teaching and learning, and research.

When we explore meta-theories surrounding why psychotherapy and counselling work, first we see that clients need a plausible explanation to account for their symptoms and experiences. Second, they need a 'road map' to orientate themselves, to see how best they can address their trauma experiences. *Breaking Free* is an excellent road map – a well-written, well-structured and robust resource for survivors, mental health workers, counsellors, psychotherapists and psychologists working in the field. I highly recommend it.

Dr Derek Farrell, CPsychol, PhD, CSi, AFBPsS
Principal Lecturer in Psychology, University of Worcester,
President of EMDR UK and Ireland; Vice-president of EMDR
Europe, President of Trauma Aid Europe, BPS Chartered
Psychologist, EMDR Europe Accredited Trainer and Consultant
and BABCP Accredited Cognitive Behavioural Psychotherapist
www.colloquy.me.uk @DPatrickF

Preface

We first met in 1983 when training to be clinical psychologists at the University of Leeds. During our training, the words 'child sexual abuse' were hardly mentioned – certainly not in relation to adults who were experiencing psychological problems. After qualifying as clinical psychologists, we both took up posts with Wakefield Health Authority working with adults (referred by GPs, psychiatrists and other professionals) who were experiencing emotional difficulties or problems coping with their lives. These clients came to us with many different problems – including depression, anxiety, eating disorders, sexual and relationship problems, phobias and self-harm – but as we talked with them, many began to disclose that they had been sexually abused as children or young people, and we discovered early abuse was a major contributor to their current difficulties.

At first, we worked individually with clients who had been sexually abused, and then in 1987 we set up our first survivors' therapy group. Group work offered a space in which the survivors were able to share their problems and experiences with others who were in a similar position, to help and encourage each other and to set up long-lasting support networks and friendships.

A psychology service was set up in Wakefield for survivors, comprising a regular programme of survivors' groups as well as individual work with people who had been sexually abused as children or young people. The groups met weekly for between 15 and 20 weeks and then continued to meet weekly as self-help/support groups. These therapy groups offered survivors a safe place in which they were able to share the pain of their experiences, work through their feelings and begin to resolve their problems.

The number of survivors on the waiting list for psychology services was growing, as more and more people became brave enough to disclose that they had been sexually abused. We decided to write a booklet on child sexual abuse to help and encourage the survivors who were waiting for therapy. Some of the former members of the survivors' groups were keen to help by contributing the writing they had produced as part of their own therapy.

The booklet soon expanded into a book, and ACT (Abuse – Counselling and Training), an action group of Wakefield survivors committed to helping other survivors and working towards the prevention of sexual abuse, was founded. Over the years, the original members of ACT have spread their wings and developed fulfilling lives for themselves. ACT was superseded by Moving On, a support and discussion group for survivors who had completed therapy in the psychology service.

There are millions of survivors of child sexual abuse in the UK. Many survivors have simply never had the opportunity to talk about what happened to them as children, and how their lives have been affected by the abuse. For this reason, we wrote this book to break the collective silence: to share what we have learnt and reach out to all people who have been sexually abused as children or young people. We hope our endeavours will go some way to mitigating the isolation experienced by some adult survivors, and help them take their first steps in breaking free from the past. We would emphasize that this book is by no means intended as an alternative to professional help; we simply hope it will give survivors confidence to seek the help they deserve.

This book expresses our deeply held belief in the power of human beings to survive, heal and grow. Had it not been for the courage of those Wakefield survivors who were prepared to share their experiences with us and contribute their writings, this book would not exist. All the events and people described here are real. Although the names have been changed for legal reasons or to protect family members, this is not because the survivors are ashamed. **Indeed, they know the responsibility for child sexual abuse always lies with the abuser, never with the abused child.**

What's new in the 2018 edition?

- Since *Breaking Free* was first written, I have learnt a lot more about the complexity surrounding the consequences of child sexual abuse, and how advances in our understanding can inform new ways to help survivors overcome the long-term difficulties. Child sexual abuse is a traumatic event, usually a series of traumatic events, and this updated edition emphasizes the impact the effects of trauma have on the lives of survivors. The book now includes more information about the symptoms of trauma and post-traumatic stress disorder, including dissociation, nightmares, hyperarousal and flashbacks. A possible cause of trauma-based hallucinations is discussed, together with a simple and effective way to manage them. EMDR (eye movement desensitization and reprocessing) therapy is described and recommended, together with trauma-focused cognitive behavioural therapy (CBT), as an effective treatment for symptoms resulting from the trauma of sexual abuse.

- Information has been updated on the prevalence, prevention and reporting of sexual abuse, the contemporary research on sexual abuse, and the resources available to adult survivors.

- In order to reflect advances in societal understanding around sexual abuse, I have made the book more inclusive by updating the language used in relation to sex and gender, and by referring to the diverse types of abuse, abusers and grooming techniques that have been uncovered and publicized in recent years. These include abuse by celebrities and football coaches, child sexual exploitation by gangs in many of our cities, grooming via social media and the internet, and the effects of unprecedented internet access to sexual activity and child pornography.

- The first chapter encourages survivors to find appropriate ways to keep themselves safe. A new appendix – Appendix 1 – provides information on how survivors can feel more in control by learning how to manage panic attacks and how to reduce their anxiety by breathing properly.

- There is now a plethora of books that describe the horrific details of the acts involved in sexual abuse and the consequent years of distress endured by individual survivors. By comparison, the emphasis of the *Breaking Free* books has always been on how to understand and *overcome* the problems caused by childhood sexual abuse. The original Chapter 2, 'Survivors speak out', has been moved to form Appendix 2 so interested readers can still learn about the backgrounds of some of the founding contributors. The main body of the book is now focused on recovery. It is my firmly held belief that, with the right support, it is possible for survivors to fully recover and live their lives unencumbered by the shadow of abuse.

Kay Toon

Acknowledgements

The ideas in this book have developed from our work with the survivors of childhood sexual abuse who were brave enough to share their experiences with us and who have struggled to overcome their problems and break free from the pain, guilt and powerlessness they felt. We would like to express our respect for these survivors and our thanks for the knowledge we have gained by working with them. We would especially like to thank all the survivors who have contributed their writings to this book. We would like to thank Margaret Ainscough, Chris Bethlehem, Alistair Cant, Sharon Jackson, Diane Carole, Chris Leach, Jon Fraise, Bryn Thomas and especially Andrew Lister for helping us, in different ways, through the process of writing the original *Breaking Free*.

Our special thanks to Erika Trueman for contributing her personal story to the book and for all her hours of typing and retyping, and to members of ACT for their unfailing enthusiasm and support for this project.

Carolyn Ainscough* and Kay Toon
Chartered Clinical Psychologists

Acknowledgements for this edition

I have been further assisted in the writing of this new edition by Annette Morris, Anna Keagan, Louisa Cahill, Jerry Hardman-Jones, Diane Carole, Faye Carole, Cath Malone, Ros Ramsden and Phil Mitchell.

---

* Carolyn died in 2000.

Part 1
SEXUAL ABUSE CHANGES LIVES

1

Survival and recovery: the journey begins

Now I feel more powerful. I'm going to take care of this power and nurture it and I'm going to take charge of my life. I'm going to get out of this mess. I can see a different life. I can smell a better future. I'm not frightened any more. I'm breaking free.
Lizzie

Until recently, the sexual abuse of a child was thought to be a terrible but uncommon event. Survivors of abuse who were brave enough to speak out were often not believed. Even when they were believed, there was frequently no further action taken. The widespread sexual abuse of children and young people is by no means a new problem, however. Generations of children have been sexually abused in secret and have remained silent.

Since the 1980s, there has been an increasing awareness of child sexual abuse owing to coverage in a variety of media outlets: television and radio, books, newspapers and magazines and, more recently, a range of social media platforms. The focus was initially on the individual abuse of children in their homes or by people known to them. More recently, the media have publicized organized abuse within institutions, the sexual exploitation of children and young people by street gangs in our cities, and decades of abuse by celebrities, politicians, priests and others who inhabit positions of power. At the end of 2016, professional footballers began to come forward to talk about being sexually abused by football coaches when they were young men; there are now at least 21 police forces investigating this widespread abuse. The wide availability of internet and social media outlets has meant that more ways of grooming and gaining access to children and young people have created more opportunities for abusers to manipulate potential victims.

As more and more survivors dare to speak out, it has become clear that vast numbers of people were sexually abused as children.

Many survivors have carried the secret of their abuse to the grave; others still carry the burden of that secret and suffer in silence. The collective shame and secrecy that surround sexual abuse and keep people silent make it difficult to estimate the number of people who have been sexually abused. Only 1 in 8 victims of sexual abuse comes to the attention of statutory authorities. For this reason, we may never know the true extent of the problem. What is indisputable, however, is that society can no longer turn a blind eye to the distress of vulnerable children.

Although the results of research studies vary, it is generally believed that *at least* 1 in 10 people has been sexually abused as a child – probably 1 in 4 girls and 1 in 8 boys. Even at the lower estimate of 10 per cent, this means there are currently more than a million sexually abused children in England alone. The most conservative estimates indicate that sexual abuse affects large numbers of people and it is a global problem occurring in every country, race, culture and class (worldwide average prevalence figures indicate 18–20 per cent of females and 8–10 per cent of males have been sexually abused as children). This means that there are many millions of people alive today who were sexually abused as children or young people and are living with the consequences.

Now that survivors of child sexual abuse are learning they are not alone, they are reclaiming their own power and self-respect. In speaking out about their experiences, survivors are beginning the journey of breaking free from their past.

Who is this book for?

This book is primarily a self-help book for adult survivors of childhood sexual abuse. It is for people who know they have been sexually abused as children, even if the memories are not complete. If you do not remember being sexually abused but are seeking an explanation for your current problems, please be aware that it is not possible to diagnose a past history of sexual abuse from current problems and symptoms. This book cannot tell you whether you have been sexually abused or not.

Childhood sexual abuse wreaks damaging, sometimes catastrophic, effects on children and young people. If they do not receive help and support at the right time, the abuse can continue to have consequences throughout their adult lives. This book contains information about child sexual abuse and how it affects both the abused child and the adult survivor. With its focus on recovery, *Breaking Free* goes further in suggesting practical ways in which survivors can begin to overcome these difficulties. The emphasis remains firmly on how it is possible to break free from the abuse and lead a fulfilling life free from its shadow.

The book can also be helpful to survivors of physical and emotional abuse given that many of the psychological processes and consequences are similar. We hope that friends and relatives of survivors, and people working in the caring professions, will also read this book and gain some insight into the problems that survivors face, and how to best support survivors in overcoming them. Ultimately, however, we address and dedicate this book to you, the survivor.

Sexual abuse

We use the term 'sexual abuse' to mean any kind of sexual behaviour by an adult with a child or young person or any unwanted or inappropriate sexual behaviour by another child who has some form of power over them. Contact abuse (where there is physical contact with the abuser) includes types of penetration such as sexual intercourse, oral sex, anal intercourse, inserting objects into the child's body, or non-penetrative acts such being touched in a sexual way or being persuaded to masturbate someone. Sexual abuse does not always involve physical contact. Non-contact abuse includes being made to watch other people's sexual behaviour, being forced to look at sexual photographs or videos or being groomed to perform sexual acts over the internet. Sexual abuse can occur in person, via technology or both – social media can be used to groom a child into contact abuse, for example.

Sexual abuse includes abuse by one person, a number of different individuals or groups of people. Child sexual exploitation is a form of sexual abuse in which children and young people are given some kind of reward (gifts, money, affection, drugs, alcohol) for being manipulated into sexual activities with the perpetrators, who usually work together in groups or gangs, although individuals can also sexually exploit young people. The perpetrators of sexual exploitation usually seek to gain financial rewards or increased status from the abuse, rather than sexual gratification or power as in other forms of sexual abuse.

Even when sexual activity with a child or young person appears consensual, it is *still sexual abuse*. Similarly, the abuse may have happened only once or many times over a number of years. It may still be happening.

Survivors

We use the word 'survivors' to refer to people who have been sexually abused as children and young people. The abuse may have continued into adulthood and may still be ongoing, but this book is primarily for anyone whose sexual abuse *started* when they were a child or young person. Disabled children are at high risk of being sexually abused.

Survivors can be of any sex or gender and can come from any religious or ethnic background or any walk of life. Wakefield survivors include teachers, stay-at-home mums, police officers, radiographers, health visitors, managers, lorry drivers, single parents, unemployed individuals, nurses, driving instructors, domestics, caterers, clerical workers and business people.

Survivors have had to find ways of surviving the trauma of sexual abuse but, with the help of this book, we hope they will go beyond simply surviving to living a fuller and happier life.

Abusers (or perpetrators)

Abusers can be of any age, sex or gender. The majority of abusers or perpetrators (at least 80 per cent) are men, but many male or female survivors were abused by women (women perpetrators are more likely to abuse boys than girls). An abuser is anyone who has sexually abused a child or young person. This could be a father, mother, brother, other family member, friend, person in authority, acquaintance, another child or a stranger. It is important to be aware that abusers can also be other children who control the victim because they are older, stronger and more powerful, have responsibility for the child or are trusted by the child. Perhaps a third of abusers are juveniles; some of these may be boyfriends or girlfriends who use the relationship to coerce the young person into unwanted or inappropriate sexual activity.

Abusers can work alone or with other perpetrators. Networks of people and large institutions have been involved in the widespread abuse of vulnerable children and young people, including the Church, children's homes, residential schools and gangs of people working together. A report from the office of the Children's Commissioner found there were 2,400 victims of gangs in just over a year in 2010/2011. In recent years, terrible scandals have been uncovered instances of celebrities having abused countless children and young people over several decades. There have been many allegations of child sexual abuse by politicians and other people in powerful positions.

The sexual abuse of children is a crime, and people who are involved in any kind of sexual acts with children are criminals.

About this book

This book is for men and women who have been sexually abused, in any way, as children or young people, by male or female abusers. It is intended to help you think anew about your experiences and feelings and begin to work through your problems. Survivors who have been in therapy in Wakefield, as individuals or in our therapy groups, describe the problems they have had since being abused, and share with you the ways they have found to overcome these difficulties. Each survivor has had his or her own personal struggle, but all have been helped by sharing their experiences with other survivors and gaining their understanding and support. Writing has been part of the healing process, and through this writing they extend their understanding and support to you.

The book is divided into five parts.

Part 1, 'Sexual abuse changes lives', helps prepare you for the journey ahead, including encouraging you to find ways to keep yourself safe. The damaging consequences of childhood sexual abuse on children and adults are described and linked to the traumatic experiences of abuse. This is to illustrate how your problems may be a direct result of the abuse and not because that's just how you are or because there is something inherently wrong with you.

Part 2 'It must have been my fault', considers the feelings of guilt and shame that survivors experience. We look at the common questions that survivors try to answer: 'Why did it happen to me?' and 'Why didn't I tell?' The focus is on understanding *why* survivors feel guilty, so they can move on by challenging and changing the beliefs associated with guilt and shame. We also look at the signs or cries for help that children may show when they are being abused, how these can be misinterpreted as 'bad' or difficult behaviour, and what can happen when people disclose that they have been sexually abused.

Part 3, 'Tackling the problems' looks at some of the common problems experienced by survivors of sexual abuse and suggests ways to deal with those difficulties. It includes chapters on coping with extreme emotions, anxiety and trauma, depression, eating problems and sexual problems.

In Part 4, 'Feelings towards others', we look at the difficulties survivors may experience in their relationships with children, mothers and abusers.

Part 5, 'Breaking free', describes how survivors *can* overcome the problems, including information about how you can access psychotherapy, and Wakefield survivors write about what has helped them. We also look at ways of working towards the prevention of further sexual abuse. In Chapter 17, 'The journey continues', six of the survivors who contributed to the first edition of this book write about their lives seven years on.

Appendix 1, 'Keeping safe, how to breathe properly and how to manage panic attacks', provides information to help you take control of your anxiety and panic attacks.

Appendix 2, 'Survivors speak out', contains accounts by six of the Wakefield survivors of their own experiences of abuse and the ways in which the abuse has disrupted their lives.

This book is a first step towards healing, rather than a final solution. We hope that it will give you the confidence to break free from your past by sharing your experiences with others, contacting other survivors of sexual abuse and going for professional help. 'Sources of help', at the back of the book, can direct you regarding how to find a therapist, contact a helpline or get advice about child protection. The damaging consequences of sexual abuse *can* be overcome.

How to use this book

You will gain most benefit from this book if you read through the chapters slowly in the order they appear, completing the exercises in each chapter, if you feel able, before moving on to the next one.

The chapters build on each other and follow the sequence we have found to be most helpful for survivors of sexual abuse. It is particularly important to read Part 2 on guilt and self-blame and do the exercises in it before trying to deal with the more specific problems in the rest of the book. Some people prefer to just read through the book first and then return to the exercises, or move on to the more detailed exercises in the *Breaking Free Workbook*.

The final chapter, Chapter 17, 'The journey continues', contains accounts of how six of the contributors to the original book are doing, seven years after the end of therapy. If you are struggling to believe that it is possible to overcome the problems resulting from child abuse, you may want to read that chapter first, to see the progress made by these survivors (they are all genuine accounts).

GETTING SUPPORT AND KEEPING SAFE

If you feel overwhelmed by your emotions or have panic attacks, it is important that you find ways to manage your feelings and keep safe before you read any material that will trigger extreme emotions or before you do the exercises in this book. There are many techniques you can learn to help you soothe yourself and feel more in control of your emotions. Appendix 1 shows you how to breathe properly, and this is a really useful way for you to help yourself feel calmer – this is something you can practise wherever you are. Appendix 1 also teaches you how to take control of panic attacks, instead of the fear of panic attacks controlling you and your lifestyle. If you sometimes have the terrifying experience of seeing your abuser when he or she is not actually there (trauma-based hallucinations), it will help you feel more in control if you learn the simple technique for managing hallucinations described in Chapter 8.

You will need time to take in what you have read and deal with your emotional reactions. You may find some of this book upsetting. Don't try to push your feelings away. Accept your emotions and allow yourself to cry or feel angry. Set aside time to read the book and read it in a place where you feel safe and comfortable. It is not a book you can read casually in a spare moment. If possible, try to find someone you trust who will support you and talk with you about how you are feeling while you are reading this book. Getting help and support from others is a useful and practical way to deal with your problems, not a sign of weakness and failure. If you start to feel overwhelmed by feelings and memories, you might benefit from taking a break from the book until you feel calmer and more settled. You could also try phoning one of the helplines or contacting a therapist (see 'Sources of help' at the back of the book). Many survivors have found it helpful to work through this book or the *Breaking Free Workbook* with the help of a therapist. The *Breaking Free Workbook* contains suggestions in the first chapter about how to keep a safe emotional distance from the material while you are working on the sexual abuse. The *Workbook* also has chapters on coping with emotions, flashbacks and hallucinations, and managing triggers. Indeed, you may find helpful to learn some of these techniques before you read this book.

WRITING

Most of the chapters in this book contain exercises, many of which ask you to write about your feelings and experiences. You could write on paper or in a notebook, or you could type your responses into a private file on your computer, tablet or smartphone. Many Wakefield survivors have found that writing played a very important part in their recovery, and they describe in Chapter 15, 'Overcoming the problems', how it has helped them.

Some survivors find the idea of writing very threatening and feel that it will not be helpful, but writing down what you remember and feel can make the reality of what has happened to you very clear. Although this can be painful, it can also be a step towards dealing with the past. Writing can trigger memories and feelings that have been blocked off, and this can be frightening – although it can also be very useful in the healing process.

> At first when I wrote things, I always tore them up or burnt them immediately. I was pleased when I could read through them again. I'd pushed it all down inside me. I started writing down all the things I couldn't cope with or talk about. **Lucy**

> I didn't know what to expect and when I first started writing things down I felt OK. Later I was getting flashbacks and bad memories were returning, but when the writing was complete I felt it had been very beneficial for me. **Anthony**

Writing isn't the same as just thinking things out. Many survivors get access to their memories and feelings and begin to understand themselves better once they begin to write. If you have trouble writing, get someone you trust to write it down for you or say it out loud and record it for yourself on your smartphone or other device.

> I'm not sure what to put down. I just write whatever comes into my mind at the time. I only remembered where I'd been abused when I'd written it down. There are quite a few things I've remembered this way. **Mavis**

> I wouldn't have believed how writing it down could have helped so much – it was incredible. I could see it much more in black and white. Seeing it written down you think, 'Yes, that's how I feel.' Without writing, you don't always recognize exactly how you feel. **Jocelyn**

Spelling, grammar and style don't matter – the education of many survivors has suffered because of abuse during childhood. Remember, it is your thoughts and feelings that are important and they need to be written down.

After you have finished a piece of writing, it can be even more helpful to read your responses out loud to yourself, in private. Listening to your own written responses, rather than just reading them in your head, allows your brain to process them via different neural pathways and can sometimes allow greater understanding or insights.

The writing is for your benefit; it is not necessary for anyone else to read it. If you are worried that someone else might find your writing, keep it in a safe place or leave it in a sealed envelope with someone you trust; make sure any computer files are secure. Writing can also be a good way to communicate your experiences and feelings to other people without having to talk, so you may *want* to share your writing with someone else.

Sharing your writing also helps to break the secrecy of your abuse. Some people struggle to write or use words, so it may be easier for them to use alternative methods to express themselves, such as drawing, painting, sculpting or using art materials in other creative ways. One survivor used dance as a way to explore and express her emotions, and to help her process the work we had done in therapy sessions. If you prefer talking to writing, talking to an empty chair or to a cushion instead of writing down your answers in the exercises may be the best way for you.

The healing process

It *is* possible to break free from the damaging effects of childhood sexual abuse, but this can take time. You may have had problems over many years and they won't just disappear overnight. Many people try to cope with sexual abuse by pushing away their memories and feelings. This is one of the few ways in which children are able to cope, but as an adult this strategy has disadvantages. It doesn't work completely and it doesn't last. Some survivors automatically cut off from bad memories – this is called dissociation (there is more information on 'dissociation' in Chapter 7, 'Buried feelings'). The underlying bad feelings and memories that have been consciously or unconsciously pushed away can flood back when triggered by everyday events and leave the survivor feeling distressed and out of control.

It is usually necessary to deal with the underlying problem, the impact of the sexual abuse itself, before the survivor's current symptoms and difficulties can be resolved. Dealing with sexual abuse is not about wiping out the past – you can never do that. Neither is it about blocking off the past by burying your feelings or building a wall to keep the memories away – that is usually only a temporary solution. Rather, it is about dealing with the way the abuse has affected your life and the way you feel about yourself. You will never be able to forget the abuse happened, but you will be able to release your feelings of guilt and reclaim your power and self-respect.

This book aims to help you deal with the underlying problem by facing up to your memories and feelings and challenging your long-held beliefs. This is what Claire said about her experience in group therapy:

> Things seemed to get worse as they were stirred up and brought up to the surface, but then it got better. You get a bit worse before you get better and when that happens you get frightened and feel you want to pack it in, but suddenly you change. Then you look at yourself and see the difference. **Claire**

You may feel that reading this book is making you feel worse at first as you begin to face the pain of your past, but remember, this is a normal part of the healing process. Carry on when you feel able to and you should begin to feel better. If you begin to feel distressed, take some time out from reading and look after yourself. Try to relax and ask for support from other people. Do something you enjoy, such as having a bath, going for a walk, talking to friends or listening to music. Try the breathing exercises in Appendix 1. When you feel ready, return to the book and carry on reading.

Kate attended a survivors' group. After time and effort spent working through her bad feelings and difficulties, this is what she has to say:

> Maybe I did lose my childhood, but I managed to find the 'little girl in me' and now look after her. I feel so great now. No longer is there an ugly monster looming at the back of my mind, rearing its ugly head and constantly affecting my life. Now I am in control. **Kate**

This book could be the first step in helping you to regain your own power and strength. Meeting other survivors or getting further help from an experienced therapist could be the next. You can also continue the process of working on your problems with the *Breaking Free Workbook*, which develops the ideas in *Breaking Free* by setting out practical exercises for working step by step on the problems resulting from child abuse.

2

The impact of child sexual abuse

Many thousands of children and young people are sexually abused every year, and each survivor's experience is different from everybody else's. Children and young people are abused in many different ways, by different types of people and for different lengths of time. Linking these survivors' experiences, however, is the pain they have suffered, the damage that has been done to them and the ways in which they have struggled to survive. Survivors reading this book will be at different stages of working through their problems, but we hope each of you can find courage and hope, and a way of breaking free of the difficulties in your life.

Appendix 2, 'Survivors speak out', contains the stories of some of the Wakefield survivors who contributed to this book. In their own words, the survivors describe the abuse they experienced as children, and the problems the abuse caused in their lives both as children and as adults. The stories can be very distressing in themselves, and they can also trigger bad memories and feelings about any abuse you may have experienced. Appendix 2 is for readers who want to learn more about the background of some of the survivors who have contributed to this book, but please do not feel that you *should* read it. There are now many books in existence that describe the horrible experiences suffered by survivors of sexual abuse and their personal stories of recovery. The emphasis in this book is to provide suggestions on how to understand and *recover from* the consequences of sexual abuse, rather than describe the abuse history itself.

The aim of this chapter is to help you make connections between the abuse you experienced as a child or young person and the many ways this has affected your life up until now. The way you feel, the way you think, how you behave, your physical symptoms, what you do to cope, your relationships with people, your personality, and how you feel about yourself and your own body, may all have been affected by the childhood abuse. Realizing you have problems now because something very bad has happened to you, rather than because there is something wrong with you, may help you be a little kinder to yourself.

Understanding how you have been affected, and how these changes are the long-term consequences of sexual abuse, is an important step in moving on from the abuse. Our work, over many years, with survivors has convinced us that it is possible for people to overcome their problems and move on from the impact of childhood sexual abuse. The following chapters encourage you to continue your own journey towards breaking free from the abuse by tackling these problems and working on the underlying issues, including feeling guilty and powerless.

Feeling different

We have learnt about the consequences of sexual abuse from our clients who were survivors of abuse, and particularly from the survivors who attended our therapy groups. At the end of the first meeting of a survivors' group, the group members usually say that they feel relieved and surprised to find that they are not alone. They find other people in the group have had similar experiences and have suffered similar problems as a result of being sexually abused. By the beginning of the second meeting, however, the survivors have usually managed to find some reason why they think they are still different from the rest of the group, and why they shouldn't be in the group or don't deserve to receive help:

- 'I was only abused once.'
- 'I was abused by a woman.'
- 'I had lots of abusers.'
- 'The abuser didn't have intercourse with me.'
- 'I was a teenager when the abuse started.'
- 'It started when I was a baby.'
- 'My abuser was another child.'
- 'The abuser wasn't a family member.'
- 'I enjoyed the sexual stimulation.'
- 'I've never tried to kill myself.'
- 'My abuse was worse than theirs.'

- 'What happened to me doesn't seem as bad as what's happened to everyone else.'

Many survivors feel frightened and distressed when they see how sexual abuse has damaged other survivors. They may try to convince themselves that they haven't been as badly affected by focusing on the differences between their experiences and other people's. Survivors often feel guilty, ashamed and worthless, so emphasizing these differences may be a way of saying, 'I don't deserve to be helped.' Many survivors have felt different, or an outsider, for most of their lives.

Many children and young people are sexually abused by men (often family members). Most abusers are men, but up to 20 per cent of abusers are women. It can be difficult to accept that some women sexually abuse their own children, and this clearly has a devastating effect on the children involved. Abusers can be of any gender or sexual orientation; they can be family members, other children, friends, strangers, acquaintances or people in positions of authority.

Sexual abuse includes many different types of physical acts or may not involve physical contact at all; for example, it may be taking photos of a child in sexual poses, exposing genitals, engaging a child in phone sex or sexting, or grooming them online. Physical acts of abuse include inappropriate touching, masturbation, intercourse, oral sex and penetration with objects. The acts are different, but they are all acts of abuse. The acts involved in sexual abuse may be more extreme and involve physical violence, animals, sex with groups of people, rituals, confinement, pornography and torture. Sexual abuse can be perpetrated by one or many abusers, working separately or together. It may occur on a regular basis over many years or it may happen on only one occasion.

You may have heard, or read about, many descriptions of child sexual abuse, whether online, on the television or radio, in magazines, from people you know or in books and movies. The experiences may have been very different from each other, but they were all sexual abuse. When you hear about other people's experiences of sexual abuse, do you focus on the differences, or the similarities, between your experiences and theirs? Your story may be quite different from theirs, but if you have had an inappropriate or unwanted sexual experience as a child or young person, you have suffered abuse.

Survivors are not just affected when the abuse is actually happening to them, the consequences can continue to affect them throughout their lives. Some survivors develop serious problems in many areas of their lives and are unable to cope. Some have support and resources as children and adults, which enable them to minimize or overcome the effects of their abusive experiences. Others may appear to cope very well on the surface, but are struggling with fears and insecurities underneath. Box 1 lists the most common long-term effects of sexual abuse. How many apply to you?

Survivors frequently do not realize the extent to which they have been affected by being sexually abused.

> Before I joined a survivors' group, I felt confused – did the abuse really happen? I even thought I'd come through it unscathed; it hadn't really affected me. I was blinkered, everything has been affected, me, my personality, my sexuality, my relationships with everyone – parents/adults/friends, male and female. Who was I? Who am I? **Jocelyn**

Before Jocelyn joined a survivors' group, she felt that sometimes getting depressed, having feelings that she couldn't cope with and not liking to make close friendships were just part of her personality. She was amazed to find that the other women in the group had similar feelings and difficulties. Gradually, the patterns began to appear and she realized that her present difficulties were connected to her childhood abuse. Like Jocelyn, survivors often think:

- 'That's just the way I am.'
- 'I'm not very lovable, that's why I keep having disastrous relationships.'
- 'I'm not very clever, that's why I didn't do well at school.'
- 'I'm a loner.'
- 'I'm a weak person.'
- 'There is something wrong with me.'
- 'I'm not very nice.'
- 'I was a difficult child.'

Survivors are usually aware of the difficulties they experienced as a child because of the abuse (more on this in Chapter 5, 'Silent ways

---

Box 1 *Effects of sexual abuse*

- Fears.
- Anxiety.
- Phobias.
- Nervousness.
- Panic attacks.
- Nightmares.
- Sleep problems.
- Depression.
- Shame.
- Guilt.
- Feeling like a victim.
- Lack of self-confidence.
- Feeling different from others.
- Feeling self-conscious.
- Feeling unable to take action or change situations.
- Feeling dirty.
- Being obsessed with cleaning or washing.
- Constant worrying thoughts.
- Suicide attempts.
- Self-harming (such as slashing arms).
- Blackouts.
- Fits.
- Not remembering what has happened for hours or days (dissociating).
- Creating different identities/personalities.
- Binge-eating.
- Self-induced vomiting.
- Compulsive eating.
- Anorexia nervosa.
- No interest in sex.
- Fear of sex.
- Avoiding specific sexual activities.
- Feeling unable to say 'No' to sex.
- Being obsessed with sex.
- Aggressive sexual behaviour.
- Flashbacks (experience of reliving past traumas).
- Hearing the abuser's voice when he or she isn't there.
- Seeing the abuser when he or she isn't there (trauma-based hallucinations).

- Psychosis (hearing voices, paranoia, hallucinations).
- Confusion about sexual orientation (homosexual or heterosexual).
- Confusion about sexual identity (male or female).
- Being unable to get close to people.
- Marrying young to get away from home.
- Relationship problems.
- Unable to love, or show affection to, children.
- Excessive fear for children.
- Alcohol problems.
- Drug problems.
- Employment problems.
- Being re-victimized.
- Criminal involvement.
- Needing to be in control.
- Delinquency.
- Aggressive behaviour.
- Bullying.
- Abusing others.
- Clinging and being extremely dependent.
- Anger.
- Hostility.
- Problems communicating.
- Distrusting people.
- Working too hard.
- Difficulty in being able to judge people's trustworthiness.
- Physical/medical problems.

of telling'), but some survivors find it difficult to accept that being abused as a child can continue to affect them many years later. It may seem too fantastic, or too frightening, an idea to believe.

WHY DOES BEING SEXUALLY ABUSED AS A CHILD CONTINUE TO AFFECT SURVIVORS AFTER THE ABUSE HAS ENDED?

Finkelhor's model: four ways in which childhood sexual abuse causes problems

David Finkelhor, an American researcher, has tried to explain how sexual abuse affects children and young people, and how it also leads on to long-term problems when they become adults.

He suggests four ways in which childhood sexual abuse causes problems:

1 traumatic sexualization
2 stigmatization
3 betrayal
4 powerlessness.

The Wakefield survivors have found this model very useful in helping them understand how sexual abuse can fundamentally affect a person's life. The processes of stigmatization, betrayal and powerlessness apply equally well to people who have been physically and emotionally abused, and apply to adult rape as well. We take a closer look at this model below.

TRAUMATIC SEXUALIZATION
Children and young people usually feel frightened, confused or distressed when they are being sexually abused and may also experience physical pain. Their early experience of sexual behaviour and sexuality is traumatic and inappropriate. The physical and emotional pain involved in sexual abuse means that sex becomes associated with bad feelings. These feelings can continue into adulthood and lead to fears and phobias about sex, and a dislike or avoidance of sex, touching or intimacy. Survivors may have difficulties in becoming aroused or reaching an orgasm, and may experience 'flashbacks' to the abuse during sex.

When the abuse began, Graham was very young and he thought that these terrible experiences happened to everyone. He told us how painful, shameful and humiliating it was to be forced to have sex with his mother and her boyfriend. However, not all children and young people experience such distress when abuse first begins; part of the grooming process is to give the child something he or she wants in order to trap the child into the abusive situation. Anita had a violent alcoholic father and was happy for her mother when she remarried. Anita loved the kisses and cuddles she received from her stepfather at the beginning:

> My stepfather made a terrible fuss of me. I felt so special, I had never had attention like this before and I loved it. I threw myself at him. Every time he sat down I'd jump on his knee and throw my arms round him. He'd kiss and cuddle me and I felt so special. **Anita**

However, when the abuse progressed:

> 'And you do understand, Anita, it's because I love you so much that I do these things to you. Don't be frightened. I won't hurt you. You'll like it, I promise. I do love you.' But he did hurt me. It was horrible. He did terrible things to me and I was so frightened. **Anita**

Sometimes children and young people enjoy parts of the touching and many experience sexual pleasure and orgasm.

> My father would put his hand between my legs and rub my clitoris (I didn't know what it was then). I would always feel a great deal of shame afterwards because what he was doing felt nice. **Sandra**

When children and young people are sexually abused, they are exposed to sexual experiences that are inappropriate or too advanced for their age or level of development. They are also given confusing and incorrect messages about sexual behaviour. If they are groomed or abused via the internet, they may have seen videos that present a distorted or unrealistic view of sexual behaviours. As a result of their inappropriate sexual experiences, survivors can grow up confused about their own sexual feelings and what normal sexual behaviour is. Their sexual experience, knowledge and identity are not allowed to develop naturally. This leads to sexual difficulties in adults ranging from fears and phobias about sex, to preoccupation and obsessions with sex. Survivors, like Graham, who were abused by someone of the same sex (by many male perpetrators, as well as by his mother) may be confused about their sexual orientation.

Sexual difficulties are discussed in more detail in Chapter 11, 'Sex and sexuality'.

STIGMATIZATION

Some children and young people who are abused may believe for a time, like Graham did at the beginning, that what is happening to them is 'normal' and happens to everyone. However, at some point most victims feel there is something wrong and shameful about the abuse, even when they do not understand exactly what is happening.

The abuser may blame the child for the abuse, tell him or her to keep the abuse secret and frighten the child into silence. This secrecy makes the child feel that there is something to be guilty and ashamed about. Other people who are told, or find out, about the abuse may be shocked and blame the victim or put pressure on him or her to remain silent. These reactions add to the feeling of shame. Jane was sexually abused by her stepfather and never told anyone what was happening until she was an adult; Dorothy kept the secret of the sexual abuse by her brother all through her childhood. Although no threats were used, they felt the stigma of the abuse and knew they had to remain silent. Adult survivors often continue to keep the secret for fear of other people's reactions and because they feel ashamed.

Many survivors blame themselves for the abuse and throughout their lives feel responsible and guilty for anything bad that happens to them or to other people they know. Survivors often do not like themselves and feel different from other people. They therefore isolate themselves from people and avoid making close friendships. Graham spent much of his time secluded in his bedroom where he felt safer. Eileen was sexually abused by her uncle starting from when she was just a toddler. She has spent most of her adult life feeling dirty, disgusted, ashamed and as if she was 'unfit to be a human being'. She has never made close friends and has always felt different from other people.

The feelings of shame and guilt can lead survivors to abuse and punish themselves with drugs or alcohol, or through self-harm and suicide attempts. Dorothy was sexually abused in horrific ways by her older brother; her feelings of stigma and shame were so great that she mutilated her body with glass and razor blades and put pepper in her eyes so that she would not have to look at anyone. She also tried to kill herself. Dorothy keeps her distance from other people and feels the whole world is looking at her when she leaves the house. Graham felt ashamed and unclean, and he tried to cope with this by self-harming, abusing laxatives and cleaning his body excessively. Some survivors feel so different that they see themselves as outsiders, unable to care about what happens to them or what they do. Survivors who feel like this may start to behave in criminal or antisocial ways and end up in court or prison. Part 2 of this book focuses on how you can challenge and change the feelings of guilt and shame.

BETRAYAL

When a child is abused, especially by a relative or someone he or she knows and likes, that person betrays the child's trust. Abusers often build up trusting relationships with a child and may make him or her feel wanted and cared for before the abuse begins. They manipulate the child's trust and vulnerability, and have no regard for his or her well-being. The child may also feel betrayed by his or her mother, or other non-abusing adults, if the child is not supported or protected by them.

Anita was vulnerable; she received very little attention from her biological parents and was overwhelmed by the affection shown to her by her new stepfather. She soon trusted him, but the kissing and cuddling turned into sexual abuse; Anita's trust was betrayed.

> 'It's good, isn't it, Anita? You like this, don't you? I told you that you would, didn't I?' I was so scared I couldn't move. My body was stiff and tears were rolling down my cheeks. Yet still he seemed to be in a fantasy world believing I was really enjoying it. **Anita**

Despite Anita's tears and obvious distress, her stepfather continued to abuse her. Anita's mother also betrayed her, by failing to protect her from the abuse. Her well-being was disregarded, and she was treated abusively by the very people who were supposed to love and protect her.

Jane's stepfather also betrayed Jane's trust in her 'proper family' and her new daddy, by sexually abusing her. Graham was abused and betrayed by his mother, who also rented him out at weekends to be used as a child prostitute. Betrayal can be experienced as a feeling of loss – loss of a trusting and loving relationship, loss of a caring adult to protect you. This leads to feelings of grief and depression, or anger and hostility.

Fear of further betrayal can lead to mistrust of others and cause survivors to avoid, or feel uncomfortable in, close relationships and friendships, leaving them feeling alone and isolated. The painful sexual abuse and the betrayal by her older brother left Dorothy unable to trust other people or form intimate relationships. She described her grief and how, at 43 years of age, she had resigned herself to being alone. On the other hand, some survivors become extremely dependent and clingy with other people. Betrayal by the very people one would expect could be trusted can result in survivors having difficulties in judging how trustworthy other people are. Survivors with children may find it hard to judge who is trustworthy around their children.

Trustworthy people may be mistrusted, and trust put in those who do not merit it. Pam was sexually abused by her father as a child, she married at a young age and was physically abused by her first husband. Anita also experienced further physical and sexual abuse as an adult, including by her first husband, whom she married at 16 years to get away from home. Graham was raped by three men when a young adult. Survivors do not ask to be abused again and are not responsible for any further abuse. However, sexual abuse may leave some survivors more vulnerable to further abuse, especially if they are unable to judge trustworthiness or feel compelled to cling on to bad relationships. Relationship problems, and how to improve your relationships, are discussed in Part 4 of the book.

POWERLESSNESS

A child experiences an intense sense of powerlessness, or helplessness, when he or she is sexually abused. The child's body is touched or invaded against his or her wishes, and this may happen over and over again. The abuser manipulates the child or forces the child into the abuse. Even if the child tells someone else, the person may not believe them. The child repeatedly experiences fear and an inability to control the situation.

Many children and young people attempt in their own way to try to control the situation and stop the abuse, but their attempts are often useless. Jane sometimes managed to say 'No' to her stepfather, but he then behaved badly in the home and made her family suffer until she gave in. Jane felt no one would believe her if she tried to tell what was happening, because her stepfather appeared to others to be such a nice man who would collect pensions for the old and prescriptions for the sick, and clear snow for neighbours. She was trapped.

Anita told the school counsellor that her stepfather had 'done things to her'. The counsellor then told Anita's mother.

> My mother promised me it wouldn't happen again and that was an end to it. It wasn't mentioned again. It did stop for a couple of weeks and then one day he came in to tell me how sorry he was.

He began to cry and he put his arm round me, as he did so he began all over again. I later told my mother he had started doing things again and she said she'd make him stop. By this time, he seemed to have realized he could get away with anything and so now he didn't even wait for my mum to be out of the house before he abused me. **Anita**

Anita had nowhere to turn, she had told two adults and the abuse was still continuing; she felt totally powerless.

Pam had been unable to stop the abuse by her father despite shouting, screaming and kicking; nor could she get her mother or an officer from the National Society for the Prevention of Cruelty to Children (NSPCC) to help her. Some children, older boys especially, believe they should have been physically strong enough to stop the abuse. Feeling powerless leads some children and young people to seek out the abuser, in an attempt to feel they have some control over what is happening. Unfortunately, this results in reinforcing their belief that they are responsible for the abuse. The powerlessness experienced during sexual abuse can lead to long-term beliefs that they are unable to take action or change situations.

Survivors thus feel powerless to prevent any further abuse as adults and may end up feeling like victims all their lives. Feeling powerless also results in fears, panic attacks, anxiety, phobias and nightmares. During a panic attack, you feel completely out of control. If you have panic attacks, learn to take control of them now by reading Appendix 1.

Survivors may try to escape from their fears and feelings of powerlessness by running away from home or from school, or by withdrawing emotionally. Emotional withdrawal can take the form of depression, feeling numb, avoiding close contact with others, or living in a fantasy world. Many survivors describe having tantrums, behaving badly and how they would run away from school or home as a child. Dorothy ran away from home and truanted from school. She suffered from anxieties and nightmares and later retreated into depression, as well as having fits and blackouts. Graham ran away from home aged 9 years and slept at a railway station.

Pam suffered from nightmares, depression and agoraphobia. Pam's healing really began when she confronted her parents with the abuse by her father and was able to feel powerful and effective again. Survivors may also react to feeling powerless by attempting to take control of something and by trying to make themselves feel more powerful in some way. Eating disorders often involve a desperate attempt to exert some control, by controlling one's food intake and body weight. Some survivors try to feel more powerful by behaving aggressively or by bullying, being abusive or controlling other people.

It has been suggested that women survivors often react passively to this feeling of powerlessness, whereas male survivors frequently react by trying to exert their own power over others. If this is true, we would expect more women survivors to become anxious and depressed and more male survivors to become controlling, aggressive or abusive. Anxiety, depression and eating disorders are discussed in Part 3 of the book. Your abuser(s) have taken power away from you; Chapter 14, 'Abusers', suggests ways you can feel more powerful by taking control of your feelings towards the abusers.

Finkelhor, above, describes four processes by which childhood sexual abuse causes long-term problems, and some of these processes are also common to other types of abuse or trauma. Physical abuse by a parent can also cause a child to experience a sense of powerlessness, betrayal and stigmatization.

Trauma and post-traumatic stress disorder

Many of the symptoms and difficulties described earlier in this chapter are the direct result of experiencing a traumatic event – for example, flashbacks, nightmares, phobias, hallucinations of the abuser, dissociation and hypervigilance (feeling jumpy or alert for danger). When people experience or witness traumatic events such as accidents, assaults or other life-threatening experiences, it is normal to be very anxious and distressed, and to experience symptoms such as flashbacks, nightmares and panic attacks; as well as being physiologically highly aroused and 'jumpy'. The traumatic incident continues to feel like it is still happening now, rather than that it is over and in the past.

In time, these symptoms will fade away for many people, as the brain's own natural healing mechanism processes the traumatic experience and stores it as a memory. When this happens successfully, the person can still remember the incident, but without all the accompanying distress – so that it feels more like a memory of something bad that has happened but is now over.

Sometimes the symptoms do not go away by themselves, and, after a severe trauma, a third of people will have symptoms that persist for many years. Experiencing one incident of child sexual abuse is a trauma. Most survivors will have experienced multiple incidents of abuse. It is therefore highly probable that survivors of sexual abuse will have persisting symptoms of trauma. *Why* this happens to some people, and not others, depends on a number of factors related to the circumstances; but it is certainly not related to the person being 'weak'. *How* it happens is due to a disruption in the way the brain processes information.

During a traumatic incident, a person may feel overwhelmed, and their brain may not be able to process the incoming information (for example, images, sounds, smells and emotions) as it would a normal event. High levels of stress hormones may disrupt the part of the brain that processes memories, a bit like blowing a fuse. After a trauma, memories, feelings, images, beliefs and physical sensations relating to the event can become 'stuck' in the neural circuits in the brain because the processing has not been completed. The information is stuck at a neurological level and is frozen in time, so it feels like the event is still happening now, rather than like a memory of something that is over. It may be experienced as if a video of the event is repeatedly replaying (flashbacks); some people may be constantly fearful, angry or ashamed; others may be unable to sleep; some may be 'on edge' all the time, see the abuser when he or she isn't actually there, be unable to concentrate and have memory difficulties. These experiences may happen every day or just occasionally and are usually triggered by reminders of the event; some people therefore avoid anything that might remind them of the traumatic incidents. Most survivors of sexual abuse will have some symptoms of trauma; for many survivors, the symptoms will be severe enough to be diagnosed as post-traumatic stress disorder (PTSD).

PTSD
PTSD can develop in anyone who is exposed to traumatic events such as deliberate acts of interpersonal violence, severe accidents, disasters or military action. Many military veterans suffer from

PTSD, and it is a common, normal and debilitating response to the horrific incidents that occur in war zones. Survivors of child abuse also have horrific and traumatic experiences over which they have no control, often resulting in them also having PTSD. One in three children who have been sexually abused develops PTSD.

The criteria for a diagnosis of PTSD are:

- being exposed to a traumatic event (for example, a serious accident or child sexual abuse);
- distressing re-experiencing of symptoms (for example, flashbacks and nightmares);
- avoidance of reminders of the event;
- arousal or numbing symptoms (for example, being highly anxious or dissociating).

Look through the list of symptoms of PTSD in Box 2 and see if any apply to you. Many of you will have some of the symptoms of trauma; some of you may have enough of them to be diagnosed with PTSD.

Box 2 Symptoms of PTSD

Intrusive symptoms
- Persistently involuntarily and vividly re-experiencing the event in thoughts, images, flashbacks, recollections, physical sensations, daydreams and/or nightmares.
- Feeling upset, distressed and/or anxious in the presence of reminders of the event.

Avoidance symptoms
- Avoiding places, thoughts, conversations and/or people associated with the event.
- Problems recalling some aspects of the event.
- Losing interest in formerly enjoyable and important activities of life.
- Feeling 'removed' from other people or isolating yourself from others.
- Feeling emotionally numb.

Arousal symptoms/hyperarousal/hypervigilance
- Being on the alert for danger.
- Being jumpy and easily startled, feeling 'on edge'.
- Experiencing sleep disturbances (such as not being able to get to sleep, waking up often or having vivid dreams or nightmares).
- Difficulty concentrating.
- Irritability or angry outbursts.

ADJUSTMENT DISORDER

The impact of being traumatized by a rape or sexual assault as an older child or teenager can result in a drastic change in how you see yourself, the world and your identity. If you struggle to cope with how the assault has affected you, your set of symptoms may be called an 'adjustment disorder', that is, you are struggling to adjust to the traumatic or stressful event.

COMPLEX PTSD

Many survivors live through repeated experiences of abuse over a prolonged period of time. This often results in additional symptoms not covered by the diagnosis of PTSD, which is mostly concerned with the effects of a single trauma. This group of symptoms is some-times called complex PTSD (although this is not yet a diagnostic category).

Experiencing repeated traumatic experiences of abuse can result in problems with attachment – for example, difficulties in feeling connected to other people. Many sexually abused children are not protected when they are young and vulnerable, and do not have a consistent relationship or secure attachment to a parent or care-giver. As adults, it can be difficult for them to become attached or feel safe in relationships. A lack of consistent emotional regula-tion or soothing by a parent or caregiver when a young child is distressed can result in the child not learning how to manage his or her own emotions. As adults, they may feel very anxious, angry or distressed but do not know how to control their own feelings or soothe themselves. Many survivors then turn to external strategies, such as drugs or alcohol, to help them manage their emotions.

If you have any symptoms of trauma, PTSD or complex PTSD, please think about getting some specialist help (eye movement desensitization and reprocessing [EMDR] therapy or trauma-focused cognitive behavioural therapy [CBT]) as soon as possible – see 'Sources of help' at the back of the book).

Making the links

In accidents and disasters (natural or man-made), victims frequently experience an overwhelming sense of helplessness and, without help, this can develop into long-standing difficulties. After a dis-aster, therapy services are usually brought in to help both victims and rescuers deal with the terrifying experiences they have been through. Being sexually abused is like being involved in a disaster, a disaster that may be a one-off incident or may be repeated over many years. Survivors of sexual abuse need counselling, support and help, just as much as victims of disasters.

Being sexually abused as a child can continue to affect survivors throughout their lives. Many survivors do not realize that their present problems are linked to their past experiences. They often believe they have problems now because there is something wrong with them, rather than because they have had bad things happen to them. Experiencing hallucinations can make anyone think they are 'going mad', but research is indicating that people who have been sexually abused have a ten times higher risk of having hallucinations; this suggests that the hallucinations are a consequence of the abuse. The trauma of being sexually abused can result in symptoms that persist in time, often for many years, because the functions of the brain are disrupted during a traumatic event and processing of the experience is not completed. The experience remains alive and active instead of being processed and laid down as a memory of something in the past. Parts of the bad experience can get stuck in the brain – it's not your fault!

Survivors are damaged to different degrees by their experiences. This does not depend on what the physical acts were. A survivor who has been raped will not necessarily be more damaged than a survivor who has been inappropriately touched. The degree of damage depends on the degree of traumatic sexualization, stigmatization, betrayal and powerlessness that the child or teenager has experienced and whether they have ongoing symptoms of trauma. This in turn depends on a number of factors such as:

- how helpless/powerless/trapped or out of control the child or young person felt;
- what was said, and what threats were used;
- who the abuser was (relationship to the child, figure of authority);
- how many abusers were involved;
- whether the abuser was of the same or the opposite sex;
- what took place;
- how long the abuse went on for;

- how the child felt and how he or she interpreted what was happening;
- whether the child was otherwise happy and supported;
- how other people reacted to disclosure or discovery of the abuse;
- how old the child was.

This book aims to help you understand how your problems are linked to the sexual abuse and, most importantly, how they can be overcome. For now, just try accepting that being sexually abused will have affected you in some way. This isn't making excuses for your problems; it's a way of trying to understand them so you can resolve them. You deserve that understanding and help. No matter how small your problems are, they are worth working on; no matter how big your problems are, you can overcome them.

For many survivors, accepting the link between sexual abuse and their present difficulties can be distressing and frightening. They don't want to believe that, after all these years, the abuse is still affecting them. Accepting the link, as Jocelyn found, can also be enlightening and hopeful. Problems that could not be explained become understandable, and with understanding comes the possibility and hope of healing. Without help, these problems can continue indefinitely. With help, survivors *can* and *do* overcome these problems.

Exercises
Before doing these exercises, read the notes about writing in Chapter 1.

1 Look at the effects of sexual abuse listed in Box 1 and tick off any that apply to you. If you find doing this distressing, remember to take your time and breathe slowly and calmly (as described in Appendix 1).
2 Write an account of how you feel you have been affected as a child and an adult by being sexually abused. It is impossible to know for certain, but use what you have read in this chapter to re-examine your life and try to make the links between how the sexual abuse affected you at the time and what has happened to you since then.
3 Look at the symptoms of PTSD in Box 2. If you are struggling to cope with any of these symptoms, please think about getting

some specialist help (EMDR therapy or trauma-focused CBT) for yourself; see 'Sources of help' at the back of this book.

4 The chapter 'How the abuse has affected my life' in the *Breaking Free Workbook* contains more information and exercises on the consequences of sexual abuse.

Reference

Finkelhor, David (1986) *A Source Book in Child Sexual Abuse*. London: Sage.

Part 2
'IT MUST HAVE BEEN MY FAULT'

3

'Why me?'

Many survivors have asked themselves the question 'Why me? Why did the perpetrator choose ME to abuse?' They often answer this question by blaming themselves for what happened:

- 'I must have been flirtatious.'
- 'It must have been something bad in me that she could see.'
- 'Maybe I led him on.'
- 'I was big for my age and well developed.'
- 'It was because I was the youngest.'
- 'It was because I was the eldest.'
- 'I sat on his knee and cuddled him, and I liked it.'
- 'It's my fault because I was so quiet and shy – it wouldn't have happened if I'd been noisy and outgoing like my sister.'
- 'I must have acted like I wanted him to do it.'

Sometimes the abuser has given a reason for the abuse:

- 'It's because you don't show your feelings – I'm teaching you.'
- 'You look like your mother.'
- 'You're too friendly with your girlfriends – I'm stopping you becoming a lesbian.'
- 'I'm punishing you for being naughty.'
- 'You gave me signals that you wanted it.'

Children might well believe such excuses. In addition, as adults, survivors may never have challenged their early beliefs and continue to blame themselves for the abuse. Feeling responsible for the abuse keeps the survivor silent, and adds to the feelings of guilt and shame.

Elaine's story

Susan, Anne and Elaine are sisters. All three were sexually abused by their stepfather when they were children. At the time, each one thought she had been specially chosen to be abused; they did not realize it was happening to all of them. Susan thought she had been abused because she looked like her mother. Anne had been told by her stepfather that she was frigid and he was teaching her about love. Elaine, the youngest of the sisters, blamed herself for being so quiet and shy: 'If I'd been more confident and outgoing like Susan it wouldn't have happened.' Each girl felt she had been singled out to be abused because of her looks, her behaviour or her personality. None of them talked about what was happening to them.

When Elaine was 27, she became deeply depressed and tried to kill herself. For the first time in her life, she told Susan what had happened to her. She couldn't believe what Susan said – that it had happened to her too. When they discovered that Anne had also been abused by their stepfather, all three sisters began to look again at why it had happened to each of them. They began to think it might not have been their fault after all, and to see that it was their stepfather who was responsible for the sexual abuse. Survivors usually blame themselves for what has happened. But sexual abuse doesn't start with a child, it starts with an abuser. There is nothing special or strange about a child who is being abused. It could happen to anyone. So why does it happen to one person and not another?

Finkelhor's model: four steps before abuse occurs

In Chapter 2, we looked at David Finkelhor's model, which links the effects of early sexual abuse to ongoing difficulties. Finkelhor also studied the situations and contexts in which sexual abuse occurs and found that four things must happen before a child is abused:

1 there must a person who wants to abuse;
2 the person overcomes any inhibitions about abusing;
3 the abuser gets the child alone or in a position where he or she can be abused;
4 the abuser overcomes the child's resistance.

We will discuss each of these steps below.

THERE IS A PERSON WHO WANTS TO ABUSE
First, and most importantly, a victim must have come into contact with a person who wants to abuse a child. No child or young person

can be abused unless there is an abuser around who has access to him or her.

It is still not known why certain people want to abuse children. Some perpetrators have authoritarian and controlling personalities. They do not see children as other people, but as objects that they can use for their own benefit. An abuser may be someone who feels socially and sexually inadequate and insecure with other adults. He or she wants to abuse children and young people to get sexual gratification without risk of rejection. Some abusers are sexually aroused by children. Studies have found that some male abusers show a greater sexual response to photographic slides of children than to slides of adult women, although many child abusers are also in sexual relationships with adults. An abuser may be someone who has been sexually, emotionally or physically abused as a child or adult. He or she may try to make him- or herself feel more powerful by victimizing and taking control over someone else.

The above suggestions are ways of trying to understand *why* a person has an urge to abuse a child – they are not excuses or justifications. The abuser is still fully responsible for the abuse. We still do not know why a person becomes an abuser, but there are probably a variety of factors that combine to produce a person who wants to sexually abuse a child. What we do know is that it is not a case of a person coming into contact with a certain child and suddenly becoming an abuser. Before the abuse occurs, there is usually a period when the abuser fantasizes about what he is going to do to a child.

The abuser's desire to abuse is not created by the child – it is there before the child appears on the scene.

THE PERSON OVERCOMES INHIBITIONS ABOUT ABUSING
People who want to abuse know that it is wrong to abuse children and young people. At the very least, they know it is illegal. Before they can put their fantasies into action, they have to deal with any thoughts they may have that abusing a child is wrong.

There are a number of ways in which abusers attempt to do this. They may do something to lower any inhibitions they have, they may attempt to rationalize or justify the abuse, or they may try to normalize their behaviour and sexual interest in children. Many abusers drink alcohol before abusing. Alcohol lowers inhibitions, and after drinking alcohol, people often do things *that they already wanted to do* but might not have dared to do when sober. It has been found that in about 40 per cent of abuse cases, perpetrators have drunk alcohol before abusing, and about 50 per cent of child molesters have had issues with alcohol. Drinking alcohol does not cause people to sexually abuse a child, but if they already want to abuse, drinking alcohol or taking drugs may release their inhibitions and allow them to act out their fantasies.

Many abusers try to rationalize or justify to themselves what they are doing:

- 'I'm just loving her.'
- 'It's not intercourse so it's not abuse.'
- 'It's sex education.'
- 'He's too young to remember anyway.'
- 'I'm not hurting her.'
- 'She's a slut and wants it.'
- 'He enjoys it.'
- 'The law doesn't understand the special relationship I have with my daughter.'
- 'He's my stepson/foster son/adopted son, not my real son, so it doesn't count.'
- 'I'm keeping the family together.'
- 'I was abused and it didn't harm me.'
- 'She seduced me.'

These individuals manage to convince themselves that what they are doing is acceptable. They often justify their behaviour, in the same way, to the child they are sexually abusing, and may even convince the child that they have a good reason for behaving this way. **But whatever a perpetrator says, there is no good reason for any form of sexual abuse.** It is a criminal offence.

Sexual abuse is to satisfy the desires of the abuser; it does not benefit the child. In certain groups of people or families, the sexual abuse of children and young people may have become so common that, within the group, it is considered to be normal (which it isn't). Child pornography, although illegal in the UK, is available in the form of videos and photographs. Looking at child pornography, discussing it and exchanging it with friends can encourage people to think that it is acceptable to use children and young people for sex. In 2012, 50,000 people in the UK downloaded or shared images of child abuse. The increase in sex tourism – people going abroad specifically to have sex with children and young people – also makes child abuse seem more acceptable to people who are looking for a way to rationalize their desire to abuse children.

Organizations supporting paedophiles (people primarily sexually attracted to children) have publicly argued that sex with children should be legalized, and have made the outrageous claim that children are capable of giving informed consent to sex at the age of 4. In this context, a potential abuser can convince himself that sexually abusing a child is a form of sexual liberation, but the abuse is only for the gratification of the perpetrator and never for the benefit for the child.

Paedophiles are known to openly discuss their sexual interest in children, support each other and share images and information about the sexual abuse of children on sites on the 'Dark Web'. The Dark Web consists of sites on the public internet that are encrypted and not accessible via the usual browsers; paedophiles can access the sites with special software that also protects the paedophiles' identity. A website for paedophiles has recently been discovered with 80,000 registered users, 10,000 of them British. These sites can help 'to normalize' the abuse of children for the paedophiles who visit it and make it easier for them to begin, or continue, to sexually abuse children and young people.

Child abuse is sometimes highly organized. Abusers know each other and may abuse together either in families or in groups of friends or acquaintances. Abusers sometimes help and support each other by passing child or teenage victims on to each other, protecting each other, swapping information and helping each other get positions (for example, jobs) where they have access to children and young people. Working together like this, and accessing sites on the Dark Web, are ways of abusers trying to 'normalize' criminal and harmful behaviour. They create an environment for themselves where child sexual abuse is seen as acceptable, for the sole purpose of satisfying their own desires regardless of the cost to the victims.

THE ABUSER GETS THE CHILD ALONE

Once the potential abuser is motivated to abuse a child and has rationalized away any concerns that it is wrong, the next step is to get access to a child or teenager. For abuse to occur, the abuser must get a child or young person alone, or at least away from adults who would protect the child.

This is easy for fathers, mothers, stepfathers and other family members – bath time, bedtime or whenever the other parent is out of the house. Abusers often plan ahead to get children and young people on their own by, for example, taking the child on an outing or encouraging the mother to go out for the evening. Children may be especially at risk if one of their parents is absent or ill for a period of time, or if their mother is in hospital having a baby. The abuser is often a trusted person, a family friend or family member, so it is usually easy for him or her to get the child alone without anyone being worried or suspicious.

Other abusers work on becoming a 'trusted person' by befriending the family and gaining their confidence as well as the child's; in other words, they groom the family as well. Research has shown that the majority of abusers are known to the child, and almost half are family members.

Many children and young people may have come into contact with abusers but have not been abused because the abuser did not get the opportunity. Children who are abused are unlucky enough to have been alone with an abuser (or abusers) or away from people who could protect them.

THE ABUSER OVERCOMES THE CHILD'S RESISTANCE
The child or young person who is the target for the abuse does not come into this situation until the end. The scene has already been set. The abuser is ready to abuse as soon as the right opportunity arises or is created by him or her. Abusers only have to make sure they can overcome any resistance the child might show. It isn't difficult for abusers to make sure children do what they want. Many children are taught that adults know best and that they should do as they are told. They usually don't attempt to resist. It's very hard for a child to object to what is happening, or to disobey. The child may not even be clear that what is happening is wrong, as the abuse may start at a very early age when the child is too young to understand what is going on. The abuser may have developed a relationship with the child or young person, so the child initially trusts that what the abuser is asking

them to do is OK; this relationship may have been developed online.

Abusers make sure that children and young people do not try to resist by using persuasion ('It's our special secret') or rewards (money, sweets, gifts, praise or affection), or by getting the child sexually aroused. Making children and young people feel they are participating in the abuse in these ways can result in them feeling trapped and unable to resist, and can teach them to actively seek out the abuser themselves.

Abusers also use threats ('You'll be taken into care'), and when the abuse has happened once, this in itself can be used as a threat ('I'll tell your parents what *you* have done'). If sexting, photos or videos have been used, the abuser can threaten to show these to the child's family to get the child to comply. Physical violence may be threatened and in some cases used. Children and young people soon learn to lie still if the choice is between being sexually abused or being sexually abused and beaten up. Some children and young people are given alcohol or drugs to weaken any resistance before they are abused. The fear of getting into trouble for drinking alcohol when underage, or taking illegal substances, will help prevent the victims from telling anyone about their experiences.

In recent years it has been revealed that thousands of young people have been sexually exploited by gangs of men in several cities in the UK, and it is becoming apparent that this is happening in many more of our towns and cities.

This often starts with one man targeting a vulnerable young girl (or boy), paying her lots of attention and developing a relationship with her, so that she believes he is her 'boyfriend'. After seducing her and plying her with drugs and alcohol; he will then pass her on to a group of his friends or acquaintances who will continue to sexually exploit her. The first perpetrator may do this to gain financial reward or increased status with the gang. Her shame at what is happening, her (incorrect) belief that it is her own fault, and her fear of punishment from her parents or the police (for taking drugs and so on), result in her being trapped in the horrific situation. Although child exploitation is currently observed more frequently in girls, similar patterns can happen with young men being befriended and exploited by gangs or individuals. Boys and young men may be less likely to recognize and report sexual exploitation so the numbers of boys involved may be underestimated.

Receiving some kind of reward for sexual abuse does not mean that the child or young person is responsible; the abuser uses rewards to coerce or manipulate the child into engaging with the sexual activity. The perpetrator is always responsible for abuse whatever the child does or receives in exchange for sex.

'Why did the abuse happen to me?'

You may blame yourself by feeling you caused the abuser to abuse you, or because you think you should have stopped him or her. A child or young person does not cause abuse, an abuser does. For abuse to happen, there must be an abuser who wants to abuse and has overcome any misgivings he has about it. He must then find a place and time when he can abuse undisturbed, and frighten or persuade the child into doing anything he wants.

When Ron married Elaine's mother, he came into daily contact with three young girls. He fantasized about touching them and carefully planned how he could put his fantasies into action. One night, he had a few drinks, his wife was working a late shift and it was easy to get Elaine alone in her bedroom. Afterwards he told himself he hadn't hurt her, and she wouldn't remember anyway so he hadn't done anything wrong. He told Elaine not to tell anyone or she'd never see her mother again. Elaine hadn't been chosen because she was quiet and shy. She was abused because she was unlucky enough to find herself on her own with a man who had a desire to sexually abuse children.

As Elaine and her sisters, Susan and Anne, talked to each other, they began to realize that they had not caused their stepfather to abuse them. He was an adult who knew what he was doing was wrong. He was completely responsible.

'But I have been abused by three different people, so it must have been my fault'

Survivors who have been abused by more than one person often feel that this proves that it is something about them which caused this to happen.

I was abused by so many people that I thought I had been put on this earth to be abused. **Graham**

However, it is not unusual for survivors to have been abused by more than one person. Half the survivors in the Wakefield groups have been abused by more than one person, and research has found that nearly 50 per cent of abused women have been abused by a number of different perpetrators. Steps 3 and 4 in Finkelhor's model illustrate situations that make it more likely that a child or young person will be abused by more than one perpetrator.

- *Step 3: The abuser gets the child alone.* The child's situation may make it easy for abusers to get access to a child. The parents of Jocelyn, who we met in Chapter 2, were involved in their own problems and took little notice of Jocelyn; they also rented rooms out to lodgers. As a child and teenager, Jocelyn lived in close contact with a succession of men who lodged in her parents' house, which meant she was available to any potential abusers who came to stay and made her vulnerable to repeated abuse. Not having parents, or having parents who are regularly absent, ill or neglectful, can also increase the danger of repeated abuse because the child is left unprotected.
- *Step 4: The abuser overcomes the child's resistance.* As we discussed in Chapter 2, children and adults who have been sexually abused are often vulnerable to further abuse. Sexual abuse results in a child or young person feeling powerless and unable to protect him- or herself. It is easy for another abuser to control a child or young person who has already learnt to do as he or she is told and remain silent.

A young person who is manipulated into an inappropriate sexual relationship by a man who is part of a network of abusers becomes vulnerable to being passed around the other perpetrators in the gang. Young people are kept quiet and comply with the abusers' demands because of the guilt, shame, confusion, fear and betrayal they feel. The abusers may have given them drugs, alcohol or rewards to further lower any resistance. Some children and young people feel so helpless and have been abused so often that they begin to accept abuse as a 'normal' situation that has to be tolerated or that they have been taught to seek out.

'It must be my fault because he didn't abuse my sisters and brothers or anyone else'

Abusers do sometimes abuse just one child in a family. They often find ways of isolating that child from the rest of the family by making him or her feel different or special. The abuser might favour that child by giving special attention, treats or presents, or the abuser might blame and ill-treat that child and convince the child that he or she is bad. The abuser finds ways of making the child feel responsible for the abuse in order to manipulate the child into keeping silent. But even if you were the only victim, your abuser is still responsible for the abuse.

However, most abusers do not usually select one 'special' child to abuse and then stop. They go on abusing children and young people whenever they get the opportunity or can create an opportunity. As Elaine's story shows, sisters (and brothers) may each spend years believing they are the only one in the family who has been abused. If one person has been keeping the abuse secret, other people have probably been doing the same thing. Survivors frequently discover later in life that other family members have been abused by the same person. Thirty years after being sexually abused, Sandra discovered that three of her brothers had also been sexually abused.

> I have now learned that three of my four brothers have also been abused. So, for all those years I kept quiet, my brothers did the same. Maybe if we had shared our secret, then we may have been able to work together to end the violence that was inflicted on us. We have all had difficulties in forming lasting relationships but now we all lay the blame at our father's door. **Sandra**

Discovering that other family members have also been sexually abused can be very distressing, but it does show that one child was not specifically chosen to be abused.

> I was sexually abused by my uncle from the age of 6 or 7 (maybe earlier) and I was convinced, until the age of 21, that I was the only person he had abused. I always wondered why he chose me to abuse and presumed that it was because I was the oldest. My sister was 2 years younger and almost always in the same bed as me while the abuse took place, but I always thought she was asleep and knew nothing of it. I thought that perhaps my uncle

was under the impression that I enjoyed what was happening. I was glad when the abuse stopped. I thought he would never abuse again in case he was found out. He then went on to sexually abuse my sister and my cousin. I found out about what had happened to my sister when I was 21. Everything finally came into the open when I was 22 years old and my cousin told me about what he was doing to her. It broke my heart because I felt I could have done something earlier to prevent it happening to her in the first place. **Sonia**

In the Wakefield survivors' groups, at least 40 per cent of the women's abusers are known to have abused other children and young people. Finally, this is how one survivor now answers the question 'Why did it happen to me?'

I was young, I was vulnerable and I was in the wrong place at the wrong time. I am not ashamed of what happened. I was not to blame. **Jocelyn**

Exercises

1 We have seen that survivors usually think of reasons why they were chosen to be abused – for example, 'I was quiet and shy.' Write down any reasons why you think you might have been to blame for being abused or why you think you might have been specially chosen.

2 Abuse starts with a person who wants to abuse, not with a child. The child only comes into it at the last stage. Write down your answers to these questions (from Finkelhor's steps 3 and 4):

 • How did the abuser manage to get you on your own or in a position where he or she could abuse you?
 • How did the abuser get you to do as he or she wanted?

Finally look at your answers to question 1 again, and ask yourself whether you really are to blame for being abused.

3 You can work through this exercise, step by step, in more detail in the chapter 'Did I cause the abuse?' in the *Breaking Free Workbook*.

Reference

Finkelhor, David (1984) *Child Sexual Abuse: New theory and research*. New York: Free Press.

4

'Why didn't I tell?'

Most survivors feel ashamed and guilty about the sexual abuse they suffered as children and young people. They may feel especially guilty if it went on for many months or years. Kate was sexually abused almost every week by her father from the age of 2 years until she left home to get married at 18.

> By the time I was 12 I knew it was wrong but I still didn't tell anyone. Why didn't I stop him? It must have been my fault. **Kate**

Many adults who were sexually abused as children and young people believe they should have stopped the abuser, but how could they? A child or teenager is powerless in relation to an adult. Adults are physically more powerful than children and young people, and could resort to physical violence if necessary. Even if the abuser is the child's brother or sister, or a child of a similar age, there are many reasons why he or she does not stop the abuse.

Abusers rarely need to use physical force to coerce children into sexual relationships; they can exert power in many other ways. Children are brought up to obey and respect adults, so all adults, especially relatives, have sufficient authority to make them do whatever they want. Adults and older children are also able to manipulate the child's feelings and use threats and promises to gain access to the child's body and to keep the child quiet. If it is impossible for a child to stop the abuser him- or herself, the only way out is to tell someone else.

'Why didn't I tell?' is one of the first questions survivors ask when they come into therapy. Some survivors were abused on only one occasion, but many survivors were abused repeatedly for periods ranging from a few months to over 20 years. Repeated abuse can lead survivors to believe they must have been at least partly to blame because they 'allowed' it to carry on for so long, and did not stop the abuser themselves or tell someone else what was happening.

Why don't children tell?

If children and young people cannot stop the abuser themselves, why don't they tell someone else about the abuse? They may have no one to tell, or they may not know what to say. They may be frightened that no one will believe them, and frightened about the consequences if someone does believe them. They may feel so guilty and confused that they dare not tell anyone because they believe it is their own fault that it is happening. Box 3 lists some of the many reasons why children and young people keep the secret and continue to suffer the abuse. We will look at some of these reasons in the rest of this chapter.

Box 3 Why children don't tell

Below is a list of the reasons why survivors didn't tell when they were being abused. The words 'child' or 'children' are used here to include young people as well.

1 Who to tell?
- Parents dead, ill, absent.
- Parents involved in the abuse.
- No trustworthy adult around.
- No opportunity to talk alone with a trusted adult.
- Caregivers do not listen, too involved with their own problems.
- Frightened of parents.
- Parents discourage talk about sex.
- No friends.
- Don't know who to trust.
- No one to tell.

2 What to say?
- Child too young to talk.
- Child doesn't know how to describe what has happened.
- Child too embarrassed and ashamed to say what has happened.

3 Fears about the consequences of telling
- *Threats from the abuser.*
  - No one will believe the child.
  - The child will be put into a home or taken into care.
  - The child will not see his or her mother again.
  - The family will be split up.

- Affection and love will be withdrawn.
- Family and friends will reject the child.
- No one will want to marry him or her.
- Threatened or actual physical violence to the child, family or pets.
- Threatened or actual physical violence to other children or young people involved in the abuse.
- The abuser will kill him- or herself or be put in prison.
- *Fears concerning other people's reactions.*
  - No one will believe the child.
  - The mother will feel guilty.
  - The family will be hurt.
  - The mother/father will be upset.
  - The mother will reject the child.
  - Other people will think the child is to blame.
  - Other people will think the child is dirty, contaminated or disgusting.
  - The child will be rejected and the abuser supported.
- *Fears for the abuser.*
  - The abuser will be hurt and rejected.
  - The abuser will be put in prison.
  - The abuser will get beaten up.
  - The abuser will kill him- or herself.
- *Fears that telling won't help.*
  - Nothing will change.
  - No one can stop it.
  - Events will get out of control.
  - Fear of the unknown.
  - It might get worse.
  - The abuser is too powerful and can't be stopped.

4 The child's confusion
- *Feelings and thoughts that prevent children and young people from telling include:*
  - feelings of guilt, self-blame, shame and embarrassment;
  - confusion – 'Is it really happening?', 'Is it wrong?';
  - thinking the abuse is normal and happens to everyone;
  - not understanding what is happening;
  - believing he or she is the only one this has ever happened to;
  - feeling dirty, contaminated, polluted;
  - feeling trapped by the secrecy;

- feeling he or she is being punished and deserves it;
- hoping the abuse won't happen again;
- blocking off all memories of the abuse (consciously);
- dissociating from the abuse (automatic);
- feeling sorry for the abuser;
- not wanting to betray the abuser by telling;
- feeling it's his or her fault because of taking sweets, money, toys or other rewards from the abuser;
- feeling it's his or her fault because of taking alcohol, cigarettes or illegal drugs from the abuser;
- feeling it was his or her fault because of learning to seek out the abuser;
- believing he or she loves the abuser or the abuser loves him or her;
- enjoying the sexual stimulation;
- enjoying the affection, warmth or closeness;
- thinking, 'I didn't tell when it first happened, so how can I tell now?'

WHO TO TELL?

I didn't tell – I had no one to tell. Nobody listened or took any notice. Of course, I never said anything out loud. I cried and I always had 'tummy ache', I ran away from school, I even begged not to go out with the man who abused me, but none of these things altered anything. Circumstances stopped the abuse, not me, I couldn't stop it. **Jocelyn**

A child may be worried and distressed about the abuse he or she is suffering and decide to tell someone about it. Who can they tell? You can't just tell anyone about something you find so confusing and shameful. The only people who may be able to help are parents, a trusted adult or someone in authority.

I don't really think I would have told anyone other than my mum because the secret was so big. **Jane**

Some children and young people do tell their mothers or non-abusive caregivers when they are being abused. Other children do not have a mother or close guardian to whom they can talk about the abuse. The mother may have left home or be ill, dead or away in hospital. She may be the abuser or involved in the abuse. Mothers who are physically present may be preoccupied with their own problems or not have the time or patience to listen. Some children and young people do not have an adult with whom they have a close and confiding relationship.

> Looking back in hindsight, I know I would not and could not have told anybody. The reasons I kept quiet were very real ones. The relationship I had with my parents was not stable or loving enough to give me confidence and trust in them. They would have considered themselves and others first; what was best for me would not have crossed their minds. My father would go crazy over minor, needless things. What would he have done faced with this? My mother never listened to us properly. That stands out in my mind. When I was crying and pleading with her not to send me out one day with the abuser she said, 'Why? Don't be silly, go on, go.' Never, never listened, would ask 'Why?' and then not wait for an answer. **Jocelyn**

Even if the child or young person has a good relationship with his or her parents, there are many reasons why they might not tell them about the abuse. In some households, sex is a taboo subject and the parents are very strict so children are too frightened to talk about sex or bring up the subject of sexual abuse. Embarrassment alone prevents many young people from talking; the shame and stigma that surround sexual abuse make it a very difficult subject to talk about. Children who are being abused often withdraw into their shame, distrust people and avoid getting close to anyone in order to stop their secret from being discovered. They don't have a friend to tell.

WHAT TO SAY

Even children and young people who do have a good relationship with a trusted adult may find it impossible to tell him or her. How do you tell? What do you say? Many children are abused from a very early age, too young to talk or too young to know what is happening to them. Older children may not know how to talk about what is happening to them. They may blurt out, 'Daddy keeps touching me.' *They* know what kind of touching they mean, but the adult they are talking to may not and may assume it is tickling or some innocent form of touching.

> I never told anyone of my abuse although at one point (when I was approximately 11) I decided to do something about it because

my uncle actually tried to have intercourse with me and it was then that I could take no more. I tried to tell my mother but all that came out was that I didn't want to stay at my uncle's any more (I stayed at least once a week usually). I told her he used to come into the bathroom while I was undressed or in the bath and generally made me feel uncomfortable. I never actually revealed that he had touched me although I tried to give hints. **Sonia**

Teenagers also find it very difficult to talk about sexual abuse. They may feel too ashamed and embarrassed and not know how to introduce the subject. They may think they are old enough or big enough to stop the abuse themselves.

FEARS ABOUT THE CONSEQUENCES OF TELLING

I have often asked myself, 'Why didn't I tell anyone about my sexual abuse?' Now I can actually think of a number of reasons. I didn't tell through fear of what might, or according to my abuser, what *would* have happened. I was always being told that I'd be put into a home and that once word got around no one would ever want to have anything to do with me. More so, I would never ever have a boyfriend. According to the abuser, my mother would not want to have anything to do with me, and as I didn't have a very good relationship with my mother I didn't find this hard to believe. I do believe deep down that if I had come out with what was happening in a straightforward way to my mother the result would have been just the same. I am beginning to realize that I have been torturing myself with the question for no need at all. I only wish I had realized a lot sooner. **Joanne**

Even if a child does have a trusted adult to talk to, and does know how to describe what has been happening, he or she may still not tell because of fears about what might happen. These fears are discussed below and include threats from the abuser, fears that the child might not be believed, fears about other people's reactions, fears about what might happen to the abuser and a fear that nothing will change.

Threats from the abuser

My dad would say 'You'll be sent away and I'll be sent to jail if you tell.' Dad also said, 'It will be our secret. Mummy and Daddy will not love you any more, if you tell.' So part of my fear, why I didn't tell Mum, was because it would upset her and the family would split up. I cared about my mother and I couldn't bear to upset her. I had nobody else that I could tell at that time and I was frightened. **Lucy**

Young people of all ages fear being rejected by, or separated from, their mothers. Abusers, especially fathers and other family members, play on this fear and often tell the child it will be his or her fault if the family is split up or if the mother is upset. The child is left feeling responsible for keeping the family together and saving his or her mother from being hurt, even though it is the abuser who is wreaking harm on the family.

Graham was sexually abused by his mother. The only person who showed him any affection in his childhood was his grandmother.

> My mother always told me the police would think I was a 'dirty little bastard' if I told them and they would take me away to a children's home and I would never see grandmother again. **Graham**

The child or young person may have been told that the police already know what is happening, or that the police would blame the victim if they found out, or even that the police are involved (particularly when networks of abusers are involved). Young people being sexually exploited by gangs may have heard of incidents where the police have left victims of exploitation with the men who were abusing them. The young person then thinks there is no point in telling: it won't stop the abuse and it might get worse.

There are other threats that can be equally powerful. 'No one will want to marry you if they find out what you've been doing with me' (Joanne's abuser). Abusers often tell children that if they tell anyone they will be rejected, blamed and not believed. Kirsty's stepdad often beat her and her brothers even when they had done nothing wrong. Kirsty was therefore very frightened when he began forcing her to have sex with him and threatening her with violence if she told anyone.

> At first I was afraid to tell because he said if I told anyone I would be taken away from my mum and she wouldn't want to know me. Then came the threats and the beating, and if you knew what type of violent man he was then just the threats are enough, never mind the hitting itself. I think the reason why I couldn't

tell was that I was scared of what he would do to me and I couldn't stand the thought of being parted from my mum. **Kirsty**

Some abusers use physical violence to force their victims to have sex with them. Others threaten violence towards the child or young person, or towards other people. The abuser may threaten to beat the child's mother or brothers and sisters, or torture or kill the family pets: 'If you tell anyone what is happening, you will never see your dog again.'

Some threats are so frightening that the child is traumatized by the threat itself and may begin to hallucinate the abuser whenever he or she wants to tell someone about the abuse – see 'Hallucinations' in Chapter 8 for more information and ways of coping with trauma-based hallucinations. An abuser may even frighten the child by threatening to kill himself if the secret is revealed. Violence and threats of violence are easy ways to frighten children and young people into silence, although threats concerning the negative consequences of telling for the child or the family are more common.

Fears about other people's reactions

I knew it was all my fault and nobody would believe me. **Graham**

Young people often do not tell about the abuse because of their fears about how other people will respond. The most common fear is that they will not be believed, and this is often reinforced by the abuser. It is a child or young person's word against an adult's, and the adult may be well liked and respected in the community. In the past, even if there were trusted adults around for a child to tell, the trusted adult would probably have found it difficult to believe the child and would have had little idea what to do about it. Nowadays, there is regular coverage online, in movies and in the media of sexual abuse being uncovered in large organizations, of abuse by celebrities and of famous people speaking out about their own childhood abuse. Most people in present times are aware that child sexual abuse happens on a large scale.

Children and young people often fear that telling will hurt other people, particularly their mothers and families. They may also fear that other people will think of them as dirty and contaminated and will not want to know them any more.

I couldn't tell anyone because I was so ashamed and I was afraid I would be sent away. When we were very little, before I started school, four of us were caught comparing our genitals. Mum said if we ever did it again we'd be sent to a naughty boys and girls home. I'll never forget that. **Luke**

Their own feelings of guilt and shame cause them to fear that they will be blamed and that others will support the abuser, not them.

Fears for the abuser

Many children and young people love their abuser despite the abuse, and do not want the perpetrator to be hurt if the abuse became known. They often believe the perpetrator loves them despite the abusive behaviour. They are concerned that their mothers and families will reject and punish the abuser. Children and young people also fear that if they tell about the abuse, the abuser might be put in prison, be beaten up or even kill himself. They continue to put up with the abuse rather than put their abuser in danger.

Fears that telling won't help

The child may feel that even if he or she does tell, nothing can be done to stop the abuse.

Our family lived with my grandfather and an aunt in a very small flat. I had to share my mother's bed for the first 5 years of my life. My brother, the abuser, slept in the same bedroom as my parents and me. Because there was no space for either him or me to move out of our parents' bedroom I saw no way the abuse could stop. When bedtime came and he wanted to abuse me, I was there. There was nowhere to go. Pretending to be asleep did not help either. No way out – he said he'd kill me if I told anyone. **Ingrid**

Ingrid believed the sleeping arrangements at home made it impossible for anyone to stop her brother abusing her. Anita and Pam described how they had told their mothers and other people about the abuse but no action was taken to stop it. The feelings of powerlessness induced by the abuse can make the victim feel that no one can change the situation and stop the perpetrator.

Many children only want the abuse to be stopped and are frightened that they will make the situation worse if they do tell. They fear that they will have no control over what happens next. Other young people may be told that social services may need to separate family members and the police may be brought in. They fear that they will lose any control and have no say in what happens and that the situation could get worse. These are rational and realistic fears.

Often children and young people do not tell about the abuse because they fear the consequences. Many of these fears are rational – that they may not be believed, that they may be separated from their family and taken into care. Often, however, it is the child's *perception* of the abuser's power that stops him or her from telling. The child believes that nothing can stop the abuser, that he will punish the child and that everyone will be persuaded to believe him. The abuser uses adult authority and cunning to manipulate the young person into a sexual relationship that leaves them feeling powerless and unable to protect themselves. It is difficult for a child or young person in this situation to understand that other adults may not be powerless in relation to the abuser.

THE CHILD'S CONFUSED FEELINGS

> I wondered if what was happening was normal or if I was imagining it all. **Jane**

A child who is being abused is put in a frightening and confusing situation. They may never have heard of anything like this happening. Nobody has told them it is right, but nobody has told them it is wrong. Everyone may like and respect the person who is doing these things. It may be Daddy. They may think, like Jane, that 'Maybe it isn't happening at all, maybe I've made it up' or 'Everyone else likes him so he can't be bad – it must be me.' Children are brought up to trust adults (especially family members and friends) and to do as they are told. Abuse puts the child into a state of confusion.

> One of the main reasons why I felt that I couldn't tell anyone was that I had lived for the first 7 years of my life trusting my mum and doing as I was told. Now there was a man who was my new daddy and whom Mum said that I could trust. A major factor for me was the confusion I felt between doing what I was told by him, being obedient and not telling my mum; and being

disobedient and telling my mum. I had in the past kept secrets for my mum and she had been proud of me for doing so. Perhaps this was another secret to be kept. **Jane**

I never told anyone because I was told it was a secret and, as a trusting small child, I believed what my grandad [the abuser] said. **Polly**

Abuse often begins gradually, an affectionate cuddle progressing over weeks or years into touching, intercourse and oral sex. Children and teenagers may enjoy and encourage the initial warmth and contact but then feel frightened and guilty as the abuse progresses and they find it unpleasant or realize it is wrong. In this situation, they often feel they have encouraged the abuse. They feel they have implicated themselves and have only got what they have asked for. How can they tell when telling will mean revealing their own guilt?

When it first started, he would just push up against me. At that time I was too young to think there was something wrong. When he started touching me, I began to get a bit of sexual pleasure, not knowing that he was indecently assaulting me. It wasn't until I got to high school that I realized he was doing something wrong. I felt sick inside and guilty for letting it go on for so long. **Anthony**

If the abuse starts suddenly, children are often too frightened or stunned to say anything. They hope it won't happen again. But when it does happen again – how can they tell when they didn't tell the first time?

When it began, I was prevented from telling by the initial guilt, shame and confusion. The longer it continued, the more incriminated I felt. **Jane**

Other ways children and young people have of coping with the trauma of sexual abuse are to block out their thoughts about it, to pretend it is not happening, or to retreat into a fantasy world.

I don't remember how the abuse began, I was too young. I think it must have happened gradually, otherwise I would remember the first time. But when it became more serious, before I entered school, I needed to find a way out for me to escape the abuse. I could not physically escape, but while there was nowhere to go for my body, I could send my mind away. Again, I do not remember how it started but I clearly remember how I developed my own fantasy world in which to escape while I was being abused. This fantasy became as real to me as if I was physically there. During the abuse, I sent my mind there where I was liked by everyone and felt safe and I left my body behind to be used. Sometimes the deception was so great that I could hardly feel what was happening to me. **Katarina**

Children and young people cannot tell someone else if they have convinced themselves the abuse is not happening or if they have blocked the abuse off and do not think about it. A very common way for children and young people to cope with abuse, or any overwhelming experience where they feel helpless, is to dissociate. This is a natural process where the mind automatically cuts off from the traumatic experience to protect the child from the physical or psychological pain. Dissociation is explained further in Chapter 7, 'Buried feelings'. Children may start by deliberately blocking off the abuse by taking their mind elsewhere, but this can quickly become an automatic process. Children who have completely blocked off the abuse, or have dissociated from the abusive experiences, will not think of the abuse at all when it is not actually taking place.

I blocked off the whole thing as if it had never happened, so I never told anyone because in my mind it hadn't happened. That is until a few years ago, when I started to have flashbacks. I can't remember if I was blackmailed or threatened or told it was a secret. I somehow felt detached from it all as though I watched and it wasn't really me. **Margaret**

After the abuse has ended, many people block off the memories or dissociate, and forget all about it until something triggers off the memories again.

Some abusers give sweets, money or other rewards to the child after the abuse, and this confuses the child even more. Mary's neighbour invited her in to play with marbles. She didn't dare tell her mother about the abuse because she knew she wasn't allowed to play with marbles. Shirley was abused by a shopkeeper who gave her some sweets afterwards. She couldn't tell her mother about the abuse because she knew she shouldn't take sweets from strangers. With older children, abusers may give them alcohol, cigarettes or drugs before or after the abuse. The victims then feel the abuse must be their own fault because they accepted a reward, they also know they should not consume drugs, cigarettes or alcohol, and this also prevents them from telling anyone. Giving young people money or presents leaves them feeling confused about their role in the abuse and helps to keep them quiet about what is happening.

Abusers sometimes make sure the child or teenager becomes sexually aroused during the abuse. Children and young people who get enjoyment from the sexual stimulation often feel that, because they felt some pleasure, they encouraged the abuse and therefore cannot tell anyone. Boys often get erections during sexual abuse, either as a reflex or as a response to sexual stimulation, and this cannot be hidden from the abuser. This obvious sign of arousal makes the child or young person feel that he must be involved in, and responsible for, the abuse.

> I was already feeling isolated when the abuse started. I tried so hard to get my mother to love me but I couldn't get through to her, then here was someone giving me something yet taking so much more. All I wanted was to feel loved but instead I was used. It all started so innocently. I liked the feeling of touch and I felt equally responsible. But then he wouldn't stop. My head knew something was wrong and it didn't want this yet my body did. When he touched me I got a hard-on and wanted to touch him back. Afterwards I felt so dirty and ashamed. Feelings of shame and guilt increased, my body had let me down, betrayed me. He stole something from me. He wanted sex and he used me. I couldn't tell because I felt so filthy, so fucking guilty. **Luke**

Children and young people do not enjoy being sexually abused but they may enjoy some of the things that go with it. They may enjoy the attention or affection, especially if they get very little elsewhere. They may enjoy the physical stimulation and sexual arousal. Sexual abuse, however, involves more than affection, attention and physical stimulation. It also involves betrayal of the trust a child or young person has in an older person, the manipulation of a child's feelings and inappropriate sexual contact. The feelings of guilt and shame surrounding sexual abuse are enough to prevent most children and young people from telling anyone what is happening to them. They may feel dirty and polluted. They may feel guilty because they enjoyed the physical contact or the attention, or because they accepted money, alcohol or sweets. The child's attempt to make sense out of a situation he or she does not understand often leaves the child feeling confused, ashamed and unable to tell anyone about the abuse.

Breaking free from the guilt

You may have been feeling ashamed and guilty for many years because you have been blaming yourself for not stopping the abuse. After working through this chapter, you may begin to realize it was impossible for you to stop the abuser(s) yourself, and that there were many good reasons why you could not tell someone else about the abuse. Understanding your reasons for not telling will not make the guilt and shame disappear overnight because you have been carrying these feelings for a long time. You may understand intellectually that you could not stop the abuser but may still *feel* guilty. It can take a while for your feelings to catch up with your thoughts. Work through the exercises at the end of this chapter and do them again every time you start to blame yourself for the abuse. In time the feelings of shame and guilt will fade.

Here is Anita's description of why she didn't tell.

At the beginning, I was very young and I didn't understand what was happening. As I grew to realize things weren't right I felt more and more uncomfortable. I didn't know how to tell. At first I thought maybe I was imagining things, then I thought nobody would believe me because it was all so fantastic. Things like this just didn't happen. As I got a bit older and now knew for certain it wasn't my imagination, I wanted to tell but it had now gone on for some time, and I'd let it. At first when my stepdad cuddled and kissed me I'd longed to feel like I did. I missed my daddy so much and my mum had never been affectionate. I kissed and cuddled him back and felt really special, but when the touching started I felt uncomfortable but I couldn't tell as I felt so ashamed and guilty. I'd craved love and attention and I had finally got it so therefore I'd brought it all on myself. It was all my fault and I deserved to suffer. My mum had already had one bad marriage, now she was happy with my stepdad and I couldn't spoil everything by telling her what he was doing to me. Time went on and things got worse and worse: he'd appear from nowhere, he'd seem to be everywhere at once, every corner I turned in the house, every time I passed his hands would be touching me. Each time I was alone he'd be there and each time he'd do more and expect more and more. Every time I swore to myself it wouldn't happen again. I'd tell, but how, what could I say, where would I start? I would hurt my mum so much and probably make her hate me. He'd also started telling me I must never ever tell because no one would ever understand and lots of bad things would happen to both of us if I ever did. **Anita**

Exercises

Doing these exercises may help you deal with the feelings of guilt, self-blame and shame.

1 You may wonder why you didn't stop the abuser. Adult survivors often forget how small or powerless they were in comparison to their abuser. Doing this exercise helps you remember the differences in physical size and strength between you and the abuser at the time of the abuse. It is important when you do this exercise that you start by looking at your size when the abuse *first started*, not after it had been happening for a while.

   Find photographs of yourself and (if possible) the abuser at the time the abuse began.

   Or

   ● Draw a picture of yourself and the abuser at that time.

   Or

   ● Compare the difference in size between adults and children of the age you were when the abuse began.

   Would it be physically possible for a child to prevent a bigger child or adult from harming them? Remember that the difference wasn't just one of physical size and strength but of power and authority too.

2 Look at the list of reasons (Box 3) why children don't tell that they are being abused. Tick off any reasons that applied to you. You may be able to add to the list.

3 Write your own story of why you didn't tell anyone at the time the abuse was occurring.

4 The detailed exercises in the chapter 'Why didn't I stop the abuse?' in the *Breaking Free Workbook* may further help you challenge your old beliefs that the abuse was your fault.

5

Silent ways of telling

Chapter 4 looked at how children and young people are often unable to tell anyone when they are being sexually abused. They try to hide the dreadful secret and suffer in silence, but they are usually experiencing very strong feelings inside: feelings of fear, depression, guilt, shame, anger, confusion, helplessness and despair.

It's hard for anyone to completely hide strong emotions like these. The feelings tend to 'leak out' in some way, in changes in behaviour or moods. People may notice the changes in the child or young person, without realizing that they are signs of distress or signs that the child is being sexually abused. Instead, the child may be thought to be 'going through a phase', to be bad or even mad. We have called these signs 'silent ways of telling' because, although the child remains verbally silent about the abuse, the signs are there for anyone who is able or willing to read them. Today, with more knowledge and awareness of the prevalence of sexual abuse, we are learning to pay more attention to children's bad or strange or changed behaviour and ask 'What are they trying to say?'

> As a child I used to refuse to eat, I shut myself away and I threw myself down the stairs. I thought I was going mad and didn't deserve friends or family. I tried running away from home and I spent hours on my own crying. My head was full of questions, trying to find out what was wrong with me. I thought I wasn't normal. **Graham**

Looking back at their childhoods, the Wakefield survivors are now more able to understand their own early behaviour. Many of them had thought they were 'difficult' children but now realize they were reacting to the horror of the abuse, attempting to protect themselves and 'silently telling' about the abuse. Some of the signs children and young people show at the time they are being abused, or in the years afterwards, are shown in Box 4.

Box 4 Silent ways of telling: childhood signs of sexual abuse

The following signs suggest a child is being sexually abused (although it needs to be taken into consideration that children may be disturbed by sexual material they have accessed through the internet or social media):

- displaying too much sexual knowledge for his or her age;
- inappropriate sexual behaviour, such as tongue kissing;
- writing stories about sex or abuse;
- drawing pictures about sex or abuse;
- sexually transmitted diseases.

The following signs do not necessarily mean that a child is being sexually abused. They indicate that something is distressing the child or young person.

- Eating problems:
  - refusing to eat
  - overeating
  - compulsive eating
  - bingeing and vomiting (bulimia nervosa)
  - abusing laxatives
  - anorexia nervosa.
- Excreting problems:
  - wetting
  - bedwetting
  - retaining urine
  - excreting in inappropriate places
  - soiling
  - constipation
  - diarrhoea
  - retaining faeces
  - smearing faeces.
- Changes in behaviour or mood:
  - withdrawing from people
  - fearful of being alone with particular people
  - not making close friends
  - depression
  - anxiety
  - phobias
  - nightmares

- difficulty sleeping
- constantly tired
- suicide attempts
- obsessional behaviour or thoughts
- tantrums
- clinging to adults
- acting younger than his or her age
- running away from home
- disruptive behaviour at home
- disruptive behaviour at school
- truancy
- underachievement at school
- overachievement at school
- bullying
- fighting
- fire-setting
- aggressive or violent behaviour
- stealing
- frequent illnesses, such as stomach ache, rashes, sore genitals
- frequent 'accidents'
- self-mutilation or self-abuse, such as slashing, scratching
- alcohol/drug abuse.

It is also worth taking notice if a child or young person has money or expensive gifts that he or she cannot account for – they may have come from a perpetrator as a reward for being manipulated into sexual activity.

Some survivors have experienced only mild problems as children or only showed a few outward signs of distress, whereas others have displayed a whole collection of severe symptoms or behaviour problems. It is important to recognize that children and young people who are not victims of sexual abuse may also experience many of the difficulties described in Box 4. This list is intended only to help survivors recognize any signs they were showing in their own childhood; it is not a method of 'diagnosing' sexual abuse.

In this chapter, we will be discussing some of these signs in more detail. Many of the behaviours that abused children and young people develop to protect themselves, or release their distress, continue into adulthood. Looking at why certain childhood behaviours developed can help an adult survivor understand and accept the child he or she was then, and the person he or she is now.

EATING AND EXCRETING

Children and young people who are sexually abused experience a sense of powerlessness. Their bodies are invaded, and they are unable to protect themselves or control what is happening to them. Feeling out of control is very frightening, and people often react to this by attempting to take back control in some way. Very young children have few ways of taking control, but eating and excreting are two ways in which they can control their own bodies. Mothers of young children know all too well that battling with children over food and 'potty training' is rarely successful. Disturbances in eating and excreting are therefore obvious ways in which children can consciously or unconsciously attempt to take back control over their bodies, and show their resistance to adult authority.

The part of our nervous system that controls digestion and excretion is affected by stress, depression, fear and anxiety. Symptoms of depression and anxiety include lack of appetite, overeating, gastric symptoms, nausea, diarrhoea and constipation. Changes in eating and excreting patterns are common signs of distress.

Excretion problems

These include bedwetting, day-wetting, soiling, constipation, retaining urine and deliberately excreting in inappropriate places. All children wet and soil themselves when they are young, and remaining dry at night may only come very slowly to some children. However. assuming there is no medical reason for this, wetting and soiling that reappear after a period when the child has been dry and clean, or go on for an excessive length of time, often indicate some form of distress. When the child is being sexually abused, wetting and soiling can also be a conscious or unconscious attempt to keep the abuser away by being dirty and smelly. Adult survivors sometimes still experience instances of bedwetting. Excreting in inappropriate places may also be a way for a child to express his or her anger or distress.

> I used to soil in washbasins, on toilet seats and on the floor of the toilets in junior school. **Danny**

Eating problems

These include a refusal to eat, undereating and overeating. In teen-agers, these behaviours can develop into eating disorders such as anorexia nervosa, binge-eating and bulimia nervosa (see Chapter 10, 'Eating problems and body image'). Eating helps to blot out bad feelings and memories: as the food is swallowed down, so are the feelings. Overeating is an attempt to use eating as a way of coping with bad feelings. As with wetting and soiling, overeating can be a conscious or unconscious attempt by the child to protect him- or herself from the abuser. A girl may feel that, if she makes herself fat and unattractive, she will be left alone.

> The look of disgust on my brother's (the abuser's) face when he looked at me is still fresh in my mind. So I thought 'If he hates me fat, then maybe he will not abuse me any more if I get fatter'. So I began to eat huge amounts and gradually put on weight. It didn't stop the abuse but it increased the humiliation. **Katarina**

Not eating can be a way of attempting to regain some control (over their own bodies) but can also be an attempt at self-protec-tion – becoming too thin to be attractive, fading away, ultimately dying.

INAPPROPRIATE SEXUAL BEHAVIOUR

Young children used to have very little knowledge of sexual behav-iour unless they were inappropriately exposed to it. Children of all ages are now becoming exposed to a wide range of sexual material due to easy access to sexual images on the internet. The sexual activity that can be seen on the internet not only exposes children to sexual behaviour without context that is inappropriate to their age and developmental stage, but also provides a distorted view of sex and of people's bodies.

Children who have been abused sometimes act out what has happened to them with their toys, with other children or with adults, or illustrate it through their paintings and stories. If these behaviours are not recognized as a sign that they may be being sexually abused, the children may be blamed and thought to be rude or abusive themselves. When Kate was only 4 years old, she was caught by a teacher acting out the sexual behaviour she had experienced during the abuse with a boy of her own age, and was accused of being sexually abusive! Dorothy wrote stories and drew pictures about girls being sexually abused. Dorothy was punished for her 'bad' behaviour in drawing these rude pictures by being forbidden by her parents to spend time in her bedroom.

SUDDEN CHANGES IN BEHAVIOUR OR MOODS

When a child is being sexually abused, his or her behaviour may suddenly change. The outgoing child becomes quiet and withdrawn; the well-behaved child becomes disruptive; the easy-going child becomes sulky and moody. Adults who do not understand that this is a sign of distress may criticize or punish the child. Children can come to believe that they really are bad and therefore deserve to be abused; these feelings may continue in the adult. Some of these changes in behaviour and mood are discussed in more detail below.

WITHDRAWING

Sexual abuse by a known person is a betrayal of a child's or teenager's trust. This results in them being unable to trust other people. They keep themselves distant from other people so they cannot be hurt by anyone else.

> I was reclusive. I never wanted to play out. **Rhys**

Many survivors describe being loners as children, or getting friendly with other young people and then dropping them when the friendship started to get close.

> I would make friends quite easily but I would soon start to avoid them. I didn't want to get close to anyone. I didn't want to open up to anyone. **Jocelyn**

This barrier is also created because the child feels different from other people or feels dirty and ashamed. The child does not allow anyone to get close, in case they find out what he or she is really like or discover their secret.

> I used to lock myself away from everyone because I hated myself and thought I wasn't worth speaking to. I would spend hours alone in my room, sat on the floor at the back of my wardrobe. I felt safer being locked away. It was like my personal sanctuary. **Graham**

Withdrawing, for some children and young people, is the only way they know to cope with the trauma of their everyday lives and the burden of the secret they carry.

EMOTIONAL PROBLEMS
Many sexually abused children have symptoms of depression throughout their lives. Anxiety, phobias and a general nervousness and watchfulness may also be a consequence of being abused.

> After the abuse began I couldn't sleep without the light on, even now I need the TV or radio on to go to sleep. **Rhys**

Suicide attempts may be a way of trying to escape from the abuse and pain, or an attempt to draw attention to the situation.

> I think I was about 7 the first time I tried to kill myself. I tried to cut my wrist but the knife I chose wasn't very sharp. I didn't really want to die, I just wanted to be loved. I tried to cut my wrists about three or four times when I was at junior school. I've still got one scar although it's really faint. I think I needed to cut deeper, not just the little veins I could see under the surface. After my abuser died, I was raped by someone else. Five months later, when I was 15, I tried to hang myself. I hung myself from the window with the cord that's used to open it. The other kids laughed at me so I let myself down. **Paula**

A child's anxiety or depression may not be noticed, or he or she may receive treatment for the symptoms, without the real cause ever being uncovered. Dorothy described how she attempted suicide and received 5 years of psychiatric treatment, including many courses of electroconvulsive therapy (ECT) without anyone discovering that she had been abused. Chris was put on valium at the age of 7 because she stabbed her father when he was abusing her. Like Dorothy and Chris, some survivors may have been further abused by the mental health system. If emotional problems are not recognized or are treated inappropriately, survivors may reach adulthood believing themselves to be strange, unstable or even mad.

This sounds like a very bleak picture. However, some children and young people experience only mild emotional difficulties and heal themselves in time with the help of family and friends. Others receive supportive and appropriate help and do not carry their problems into adulthood.

DIFFICULT OR DISRUPTIVE BEHAVIOUR

Sexually abused children may show behaviour that is interpreted by other people as difficult or disruptive. The child may simply be trying to avoid being left alone with the abuser. Kate tried to avoid going out with her father (the abuser) by having screaming tantrums and pretending she was frightened of the family's car. Kate was told she was difficult and naughty. Many children and young people who have been abused see running away from home as their only way of escape; 50 per cent of runaways are victims of sexual abuse.

Tracy recalls clinging to her mother at the bus stop, and then screaming and holding on to her when she attempted to get on a bus without Tracy. The bus conductor had to help fight Tracy off. Often this kind of behaviour is interpreted as the child being clinging, demanding or wilful. Difficult behaviour is often simply an expression of the anger and upset the child feels.

> It wasn't until I was older, in my early teens, that I feel my behaviour may have been an attempt to ask for help. I remember having bad tantrums which were put down to temper (taking after my biological father who had a violent temper), but were always in a non-confrontational situation. These attempts were at home and were always ignored by all the members of the family. **Jane**

Survivors frequently continue to believe as adults that they were silly, difficult or disruptive children and teenagers. Moreover, survivors learn from this experience not to trust their own feelings. As children, their strong feelings had been disregarded or treated as trivial. As adults, survivors often keep on disregarding their feelings and dismiss feelings of anger, distress or pain with the words they had been told when young – for example, 'I'm just being silly' or 'I've always been difficult.'

AGGRESSION AND VIOLENCE

Difficult behaviour and tantrums are an outward expression of anger and distress, unlike depression, where the feelings are turned inwards. For some survivors, disruptive behaviour can turn into violence and aggression. Danny was physically and emotionally abused by his mother and stepfather.

I sniffed glue, took amphetamines and attacked people. When I was 10, I hit a classmate over the head with a half-brick. I trashed thousands of pounds' worth of property. **Danny**

Chris's story shows how anger can turn into violence and continue into adult life. Chris was abused every Sunday by her father from the age of 7 or earlier.

I ran away when I was 10. I was only out one night and I was found 16 miles away from home. I just walked and walked. But I still didn't tell anyone. I always used to be fighting at home with everyone. I had urges where all I wanted to do was kill people, get revenge. I remember loads of bad things that used to be said to me. Then I'd carry my revenge out by waiting and waiting. I always got my own back. **Chris**

Chris started getting drunk and fighting at school. Then she attacked her mother, smashing her head into the fireplace and fracturing her skull.

This sparked off care for me. I used to do all sorts. I was always in court for one thing or another. Then I got locked up on my thirteenth birthday and that was it. From then on, I went off my head. I was always in trouble and locked in a special cell. **Chris**

Chris was constantly fighting and absconding. She was sent to borstal, where she stayed for 2 years. As soon as she was let out, she attacked someone else 'to get my own back' and was sent to prison. When she was released, she stabbed someone else and was sentenced to a further 3 years in prison. Finally, Chris was sent to a secure unit for mentally disturbed offenders and was eventually released from prison aged 23. In 10 years, there had only been 5 months when she hadn't been locked up.

SCHOOL PROBLEMS

A child may show signs of sexual abuse when at school, even when there is no real problem with the school. Truancy from school is common.

I used to run away from junior school. I used to have tummy ache but my mum would still send me to school. I'd then ask to go to the toilet, I'd grab my coat and run. I can feel myself running, trying to get away, away from everything. I always thought (or maybe it's because I was always told) that I ran away because I didn't like the nuns who taught us, but now I realize it was because of the abuse. I can feel myself as a child confused and wanting to do something and not knowing what I could do. Running away was the only step I ever made towards telling or doing anything. **Jocelyn**

School may be the only place the child can let out the anger and distress felt. This can result in the child being badly behaved or disruptive, arguing with teachers or other children, and fighting.

I used to drink after playing sports for the school and I used to get drunk all the time. I was always fighting at school with anyone who stood in my way. I eventually got sent to a special school. **Chris**

In junior school I was reprimanded on several occasions for biting other children. At boarding school, I had a lot of fights in the first few years. I was often teased about my hair and clothes, and fighting was the only way I knew of defending myself. Oddly, I don't ever remember putting up a fight against the abuser. **Paula**

I played truant from school. I terrorized other children at school. I locked one teacher in a store room and spat at another one. I set fire to the girls' toilet because a male teacher came into them. Looking back, I now realize that my abuser had such a hold over me that I had to be in control. I wouldn't allow anyone else to have any power over me. I rebelled against anyone who tried to control me or pin me down. **Carla**

Bad behaviour at school also interferes with school work and gets the child a bad name. School work may get worse as the young person becomes unable to concentrate or ceases to care what happens to him or her. Survivors may grow up believing they are 'stupid' because they did not do well at school.

On the other hand, some sexually abused children and young people are excessively well behaved at school and 'clingy' with teachers, in an attempt to get the love and protection that are lacking at home. Some become overachievers at school, as they strive to escape from the pain of their emotions by concentrating their mind on work.

FREQUENT ILLNESSES

Children and young people who are being sexually abused may frequently be ill or complain of feeling unwell. Illnesses may result from sexual abuse in a direct physical sense – for example, urinary infections from the sexual activity. Illness can also be an indirect result of sexual abuse, arising from the stress and trauma of what is happening. Children commonly complain of stomach pains when no physical cause can be found. Headaches, skin problems and failure to grow properly are also reported. Jane lists a whole range of physical symptoms that she now thinks might be related to the abuse.

> Not long after I remember the abuse starting I developed tonsillitis, which ended up with me having my tonsils out. I then developed persistent earache. I was referred to the ENT clinic, which resulted in my GP telling me that it was all in my head. About this time, I was found to have a slight scoliosis and referred to the orthopaedic clinic. It was recommended that I should have very hot baths which, unfortunately, my stepfather (the abuser) oversaw. After this, apart from feeling generally lethargic and tired and being checked for anaemia on different occasions, I cannot recall any illnesses until I was 17 when the situation was bad again, mainly due to my stepdad stopping me going out with my friends. I went to my GP and told him the surface problem. He prescribed antidepressants, which I didn't take. I had also been to see my GP on a few occasions for period pains. During my radiographic training I felt unable to cope and, due to my symptoms, glandular fever was suggested although not confirmed. **Jane**

Physical well-being is closely linked to mental and emotional health. If children and young people are emotionally traumatized, they are unlikely to remain physically well.

> At about the same time as the abuse started (when I was about 4 years old) I developed asthma and eczema. I have only vague memories of the asthma but I remember it being quite bad at times. I don't remember any treatment given. However, the eczema was bad. I developed it on my wrists and the backs of my knees. I was only 5 when I had to have my tonsils out. The constant taste of pus in my mouth is still with me. The surgeon later said it was the worst case he had dealt with in years. **Ingrid**

Children and young people sometimes pretend they are ill or unwell in order to keep someone with them to protect them, or to avoid being sent to see the abuser.

FREQUENT ACCIDENTS AND SELF-ABUSE

Similarly, children and young people may hurt or injure themselves on purpose in order to protect themselves from the abuser. Mary recalls getting on her bicycle and deliberately riding it down a hill and into a lamp post. She knocked herself out and fractured her skull. She was kept in hospital to recover – where she felt safe. Lucy had an appendix operation when she was 12 years old. Although the operation was successful, her wound did not heal for 2 years. She realized later that she had been opening the wound in her sleep. While the wound remained open she was not being sexually abused.

Ingrid scratched her eczema open whenever it began to heal.

> Bedtime for me meant having bandages put all over my hands, arms and legs, and gloves put on to stop my fingernails from reaching the wounds. I even remember some nights when my hands were tied to the bedframe to stop me reaching the wounds in my sleep. I always got free and literally tore the flesh off again. I still remember the tears and the pain. My mother would sit with me and hold on to my hands for about 3 or 4 hours every night. She stayed until I was fast asleep and often then, when she tried to loosen my grip to get away from me, I woke up and she had to go through a long wait again. But because of my mother's devotion to helping me avoid scratching the wounds (which by the way I never did during the day), I was not 'available' for abuse when my brother came to bed in the same bedroom. I therefore found a way out. **Ingrid**

Self-injury and self-abuse are also expressions of self-disgust and forms of self-punishment. Children and young people who are ashamed and blame themselves for the abuse may slash themselves with knives, burn themselves, hit or smack themselves, or bang their fists or heads against a wall. Physical pain can bring temporary relief from emotional suffering.

> I used to smash my face open with my hands. I broke a glass jar and slashed all my arms and neck. I'd slash myself until the physical pain was more than the pain I felt inside. **Chris**

In her pain and anger, Fiona smashed her fist through glass windows on many occasions. At least half of the survivors we have worked with have harmed themselves in some way.

Summary

Children and young people often do not tell when they are being abused. However, they usually show signs that there is something wrong, and we have called these signs 'silent ways of telling'. Adults frequently do not understand these signs, and instead of offering help and care, they label the child as naughty, silly, difficult, stubborn, mad or bad. Outside services, such as mental health workers, are sometimes brought in to help. In the past, when sexual abuse was little understood, this sometimes resulted in further abuse and labelling of the child (as aggressive, disruptive, out of control and so on) by the system. Many survivors grow up accepting the labels, believing they are mad or bad.

Today we are becoming more sensitive to children's and young people's emotional problems and their causes. Unfortunately, today's adult survivors were rarely treated with such care when they were children. Parents, and any professional who works with children, should be trained in recognizing the signs of child abuse and what they could mean. Fortunately, many professionals, including the police, social workers and teachers, are now trained in awareness of these signs and how to support children displaying them.

Once the links have been made between the childhood behaviour and the sexual abuse, these labels can be left behind. The behaviour of sexually abused children is not mad or bad; it is simply a way of silently asking for help, or trying to cope with the strong emotions of fear, distress and anger that cannot be directly expressed. The exercises below are designed to help you look back over your childhood and understand and care for the child you were.

Exercises

1 Look at the list of childhood signs of sexual abuse in Box 4 and tick off any that you showed.
2 Make notes about what you think the adults around you thought about your behaviour as a child. Include parents, teachers, social

workers, psychologists and anyone else who is relevant. What did they say or do to you? Did they think you were distressed or think you were difficult, bad or mad?

3 Write an account of how you felt as a child or teenager and the ways in which your behaviour was affected by being abused. Try understanding and accepting the child you were, rather than judging and criticizing yourself.

4 The chapter on 'Childhood' in the *Breaking Free Workbook* may help you understand more about yourself as a child and feel more positive when you look back on yourself as a child.

6

'What happened when I did tell'

In the last two chapters, we looked at the reasons why children and young people don't tell anyone when they are being abused, and also at the silent ways they show their distress. Some of the Wakefield survivors *did* tell someone about the abuse when they were children, and they all told someone when they were adults. They often had negative reactions from people, which made them feel more ashamed and afraid to tell anyone else. Ultimately, however, someone reacted positively, enabling them to get help and take the first step by breaking the silence.

The children who tried to tell

Until recent years, very few people were aware of the sexual abuse of children, even though it was happening to children and young people everywhere. It was still a closely guarded secret. Survivors, who are now adults, sometimes tried to tell someone about their abuse at the time it was happening but they were often not believed; no one spoke about sexual abuse, and people just did not believe it happened, especially to someone they knew.

> I didn't realize it was wrong. I thought it happened to everyone. I told my school friends in conversation and they called me a liar. When they acted shocked, and were going to tell the teachers I realized it was wrong and so pretended I'd lied because I was frightened. They acted disgusted and shocked. It frightened me and I never spoke of it again to anyone. **Margaret**

Some children, like Margaret, tell other children, who do not know how to deal with it because it is outside their own experience and they are too young to be able to help. Katarina told a 7-year-old playmate who probably could not even understand what was being said to her.

The first time I remember clearly telling anyone was while my brother was still abusing me. I was about 8 years old when I told a friend of mine. For weeks, I had prepared in my mind what I was going to tell her. She was the little sister of my brother's best friend. When I did tell her about the abuse, I expected her to be shocked and show some sympathy. Because of my brother's threats, I knew the abuse was something wrong. My friend did not say she didn't believe me, she said nothing, but while I was still telling her about what was so important to me, she just shrugged her shoulders, turned and went off to play with some other children. I was in the middle of a sentence when she walked away and I felt, for the first time, the feeling of total emptiness inside me. **Katarina**

The response to children's disclosures is often that children 'make up fairy stories', 'have very active imaginations' or 'will do anything to get at their parents'. Children can make up stories, but so can adults, and adults make much better liars than children. Pam approached two trusted adults when she wanted to talk about her experiences:

I did tell someone when I was 12 years old, around the time my father raped me; I approached my mother and tried to explain what I thought she already knew. But she refused to believe it. She said I was lying – did I realize it was my father I was accusing? She said I just wanted some sympathy and attention. She threatened me and told me not to tell anybody else about this 'absurd' lie as she referred to it. I also approached my NSPCC social worker, who was no better. He tried to worm his way out of the situation by pretending it never happened. When my parents found out I'd told the NSPCC officer I got a good hiding. After that I never told anybody, I kept myself to myself. I closed myself and my thoughts within a cocoon. **Pam**

When people are told about sexual abuse, they often cannot cope with the information. They don't want to believe it is actually happening, or they don't know what to do about it. What mother wants to believe that her husband, father, sister or son is an abuser? Sometimes it is not that people *don't* believe the child, but rather that they *daren't* believe the child, because then they would have to do something about it. Pam says that her mother '*refused* to believe me'. Pam's father was a violent man and her mother was probably too frightened to stand by her daughter and against him. This is not justifying her mother's actions – Pam was left unprotected in an abusive situation – but it indicates some of the pressures her mother may have been under.

Pam also says that the NSPCC officer justified not taking any action by *'pretending* it never happened'. Doctors, teachers, psychiatrists, psychologists or anyone in the helping professions may also not want to believe that it is true. Believing may mean having to take action; rocking the boat; having to deal with the pain of the victim and the reaction of her carers; having to confront one's own pain and anger. Remember that at least 1 in 10 adults have been sexually abused as children. This includes all kinds of people – mothers, doctors, teachers, counsellors, clergy – all of whom may hear disclosures of abuse from children and young people or adults. They may disbelieve a survivor's story because they are still denying their own personal experience of being abused. As human beings, we have the ability to persuade ourselves that what we don't want to be true isn't true.

> When I was little, I did tell my sisters that I didn't like my grandad because he stuck his fingers up my bottom – at which I was smacked in the face by my sisters and told never to say it again. **Polly**

Polly's sisters did believe her, but they reacted like this because it was happening to each of them too. They'd all been told to keep it secret – Polly had broken the promise.

> It was then that my two sisters realized it was happening to all of us. One of my sisters told my stepdad what Grandad was doing to us. He came up to reassure me and promised me it would never happen to me again. He would protect me. It continued to happen. He didn't protect me. He also said that we weren't to tell my mum as it would upset her and I believed him and never mentioned it. Perhaps if I had told my mum it would never have happened again and I would have got help earlier on and not be the mess I am today. I might even have liked myself. **Polly**

Many children and young people who do manage to talk about their abuse are either not believed, like Pam and Margaret, or are believed but remain unprotected, like Polly. Some children and young people get a more positive response and are believed and protected.

Children who are not believed when they try to disclose can feel very frightened and confused. As we have seen in Chapter 4, survivors may already doubt themselves. Did it really happen? Have I made it up? Did I dream it? Being met with disbelief strengthens these doubts. Abusers often act quite normally after the abuse, 'as if nothing has happened'. This adds to the children's belief that they must be mistaken and nothing terrible has really happened. Disbelief also adds to children's feelings of helplessness and vulnerability. How can they ever stop it, if they can't get anyone to believe them? If children are not believed, they are, by implication, being accused of lying. Sometimes children are told outright that they are lying and their disclosure is met with anger and insults. The sexual abuse is therefore compounded with further abuse and the children may feel betrayed by the lack of support.

The adults who tried to tell

Even as adults, survivors may not be believed or taken seriously when they try to tell.

> The first person I told was my first husband. I don't think he thought it was true. He said, 'Well, it's past now'. He made me feel as though it was my fault for letting it happen. When I told my mum I think she felt helpless and maybe guilty. She didn't really want to know. She must have been blind not to be able to see what my dad was doing all those years. **Rachel**

Many people find it very hard to cope with a disclosure of sexual abuse, sometimes because they don't know what to do to help. Pam's parents-in-law avoided her after they were told:

> When Brian told his mum and dad about my abuse, they didn't telephone or visit for some months – they thought it couldn't happen to anybody so close to home. However, they now understand why I hate my mum and dad so much. **Pam**

Graham hoped to get help from a doctor.

> I somehow found the courage to approach my GP, who was quite unsympathetic. She said, 'I don't know what I can do' and

changed the subject. I could see a change in her facial features and I tried to hurry the end of the consultation. I was well on my way to a total breakdown and I came out even more depressed than I was when I went in. **Graham**

Although Graham did eventually get referred to a psychiatrist, he was still not given an opportunity to talk about what had happened.

Joanne was abused by her stepfather throughout her childhood. As an adult, she ensured her own children did not come into contact with him, by avoiding visiting her mother when he was around.

> Around 4 years ago, my mother asked why we didn't visit her with our children while my stepfather was in the house. At that time, he had just been released from prison after serving a sentence for abusing his natural daughter. I was so angry when my mother told me that my stepfather himself was asking as well. My anger made me tell my mother what my stepfather had been doing to me throughout my childhood. We both stayed remarkably calm under the circumstances. She looked surprised, or rather shocked, at my disclosure although I do believe she already knew and was in fact only acting shocked. The next week when we saw her she even seemed protective towards my stepfather, saying they hadn't actually had a big row over it and, to my amazement, 'He doesn't want any trouble at his time of life.' **Joanne**

Joanne's mother had believed her. Joanne believes she even knew about the abuse while it was happening. She certainly knew her stepdad had abused his natural daughter. Joanne's mother chose to support the abuser and protect her own lifestyle, leaving Joanne feeling upset and betrayed. Rhys also encountered a lack of reaction when he told his mother:

> My mother reacted as if it was nothing. I'm sure she knew because she knew my sister had been abused. **Rhys**

It is difficult for survivors to anticipate what sort of response they might get to a disclosure, as Anthony discovered:

> I found that I could not speak to anyone about the abuse for fear of no one believing me, and also being rejected by my family. I decided to be open about my abuse, years after it had happened, with people outside the family. The responses were divided – some people understood and others just didn't want to know. **Anthony**

Disclosure of sexual abuse may also be used to blackmail survivors. Lucy disclosed her childhood sexual abuse to her psychiatric nurse. He used the information to keep her silent about the sexual abuse he then inflicted on her.

Why do people react in these negative ways?

Many survivors, adults, children and young people, received negative responses when they talked about their abuse. These responses included disbelief, not being taken seriously, being believed but not protected, shock and disgust, and being ignored. People react in these negative ways because they find it hard to believe that sexual abuse really happens, they have not dealt with their own sexual abuse, or they are frightened of the consequences if they do believe and support the survivor. The emotional problems caused by sexual abuse are often made worse by these negative responses to disclosure.

> People I told often changed the subject as they didn't know how to respond. On the whole I felt I got more bad responses so I stopped telling, as it only reinforced more negative feelings about the abuse being my fault. **Luke**

Polly felt betrayed again when a trusted adult (her stepfather) failed to keep his promise to protect her from the abuser. Margaret felt guilty and ashamed after her schoolfriends' reactions of shock and disgust. Pam felt powerless when neither her mother nor her NSPCC officer responded to her cry for help. Being ignored is probably the most damaging response to a disclosure of abuse, as once again the survivor is treated as if his or her feelings and experiences do not exist or matter.

Positive responses

It is also possible to get useful and supportive responses from people. Sometimes it may take some persistence. Although Rachel had received unhelpful responses from her mother and her first husband, she was not put off from trying again.

> After I got divorced I met Paul and I thought I would tell him from the start, so that I could try and sort out my feelings. He

was really understanding and has backed me ever since. I also told Paul's mum. She was very understanding and helped me try to see things in a different light. I have also told a really good friend. She has helped me a lot and made me realize just what problems I had because of the abuse, as I always blamed my unhappiness on other things. I told my sister and she was understanding and told me she has always felt abused by my dad as well. I think other people didn't believe me in the past because they questioned whether things like this really do go on. It always happens to someone else. **Rachel**

Although Luke had had many negative responses to his disclosures he decided to confide in his partner.

When I told my partner, she was extremely supportive and understanding of the issues. She maintained that she was my partner not my counsellor. **Luke**

Rhys also felt supported when he disclosed to his partner:

After I told my girlfriend I expected her to be disgusted and not want any contact with me, but she was very concerned and to my surprise wanted to get close to me. **Rhys**

Pam was not believed when she told as a child. She went on to have an unhappy first marriage and a divorce, then she met Brian.

I didn't tell Brian about what happened to me in my childhood but, to my surprise, he told me he had already guessed what had happened to me. From his own job, he knew the symptoms, reactions and effects of abuse too well not to notice. So I spilled the beans. Since this time, he has been my mainstay. Without his support, I would have been a wreck. He is understanding, considerate, compassionate, sympathetic – everything I need. **Pam**

Graham eventually did get the response and the help he was looking for.

It just so happened that a documentary highlighting sexual abuse came on TV and they left phone lines open for anyone who had been abused. I phoned and spoke to a 38-year-old man who had been abused, which lifted me up a bit. He gave me numbers to call offering support and literature for self-help groups and that's how I eventually got referred to professionals who counsel abused men and women. **Graham**

Why tell anyone?

Many survivors have bad responses the first time they tell someone of their abuse. Why then encourage victims to tell? How will they benefit? A child or adult who does not talk about their abuse is still keeping the abuser's secret and suffering in silence. All survivors deserve the opportunity to release the heavy burden of the secret and to learn to feel better about themselves.

> When I finally did tell, I cannot describe the amount of relief I felt the next day. I was sitting quietly at my desk at work and I remember realizing that I'd actually told someone at last. I'd told my boyfriend, my husband-to-be. I marvelled at the fact that nothing terrible had happened. **Joanne**

Sharing the secret can be a first step to getting help for yourself and breaking free from the shame, guilt and pain.

> I did tell my husband and he really tries to understand. Telling the bulimia group [eating problems group] was the most useful thing for me, as now I can get help and feel that I am not going to spend the rest of my life as a victim of people who want to use me. **Shirley**

Being able to tell people who listened meant that Shirley could get help for herself and learn to deal with abusive situations in her adult life. Telling the right person can result in feelings of relief and liberation, and be a start on the path to overcoming your feelings about the past *and* your problems of today. Many survivors have received treatment for years for depression, eating problems, 'nerves' and so on, but any improvement rarely lasts without getting to the root cause.

There are many triggers that make survivors decide it is time to talk about their abuse. Some survivors decide to talk about their own abuse in order to protect other children from the abuser, or to help themselves deal with worries about their own children. Often they meet a sympathetic partner and want to tell them, so they can have an open and honest relationship. When you feel ready to talk about the abuse, be aware that, for different reasons, the person you tell may not react sympathetically. The important thing is to persevere. Nearly all the survivors we have worked with received unhelpful responses until they found someone ready to listen and to help them find a way to overcome their problems.

As survivors stop feeling ashamed and blaming themselves for the abuse, they begin talking about it to other people. Survivors are often surprised to find that many of their friends and family tell them that they too have been sexually abused, sometimes by the same abuser.

Nowadays the widespread sexual abuse of children and young people is regularly featured in the news. More people know about it; more people are ready to listen and act to protect children and help adults. There are still people around who won't listen, won't believe, will deny it, won't protect and will abuse. However, there are more and more people around who will help. Try to find one of these people.

Ingrid's story

Ingrid first told a childhood friend about the abuse and was not believed. She continued to tell different people for over 30 years until, at last, she got a sympathetic response and some help for herself.

I think I may have told some friends at school when I was still a child, but the memory of that is not clear. I know that I told my first husband before I married him when I was 17 I didn't like sex and felt that it may have had something to do with my past. He believed me, but put very little importance on the fact that I had been abused. He beat me and took me in a sexual way that showed no love, no concern, no care for me. And so during my 7-year marriage to him, my problems increased. At times I became introverted and tried to analyse my problems to find a way to solve them. I failed on my own and knew that only outside help could rid me of the memories of the past, which still haunted me. Very early on in my marriage I realized that I would get no help from my husband, so I went to my GP in Germany and told him, asking him to help me. His words were, 'Too bad, but forget about it, it's in the past.' I had trusted him completely before, but when he could not fill my need, not even see my need, I lost that trust. It took a few months for me to recover from the shock of telling someone I trusted and being brushed aside as if what caused me pain was of little importance.

My husband had many affairs, which made me feel even more inferior, and again I realized that I needed to sort out my life before I could sort out my marriage. I made an appointment with a marriage guidance counsellor, not to complain about my husband's behaviour, but to tell the female counsellor about the abuse and my consequent dislike for sex. She said it was not important what I liked or didn't like, if I wanted my husband to remain faithful I have to satisfy him in bed. She thought me silly to make such a big fuss over something so long in the past. And again I walked home feeling empty and degraded. I spoke to two more people in the medical profession, people who should have known that professional help was needed. Always the response was, 'Forget about it. He won't do it any more, so why do you worry about it?'

I had by then realized that more problems had come into existence, not only my distaste for sex. Every time I tried to tell someone who might be able to help, I also explained the effects the abuse had had on me. I got no help. Maybe I told the wrong people? I asked my brother to help me, begging my abuser to help me overcome the damage he did, by keeping out of my way. I was trying to avoid him. He didn't help me. He came to my house when he wanted to. As my first husband had become friends with him and the lover of my brother's wife (with my brother's approval) I saw him frequently. I could not tell my parents. I felt the need to protect them from the knowledge of what their son had done. But I talked to my sister, two cousins and an aunt and told them what he had done. They may have believed me, I don't know, but they looked at me in disgust and said 'He's got his faults, but he's also got his good sides, you mustn't always see bad in people. He is your brother!' I was made to feel ashamed for telling the truth.

I withdrew into myself for a while and wondered if it was worth the bother. By belittling something that I felt had destroyed the value of my life, they belittled me. One problem increased – the feeling of being worthless and of no importance. Not even my closest family seemed to care about my pain and nobody was willing to help me.

I stopped telling anybody for about 2 years after my divorce while I tried to find out who I was and what direction to take in my life. When I met my second husband and knew I was going to marry him, I told him about my childhood experiences. But he is a man who cannot talk about feelings, cannot help me because he does not understand why I have a problem. If he ever has a problem he ignores it and pretends it then goes away. He believes me but is completely unwilling to even listen to me talking about the past or my problems. So again, no help.

As my regular GP in Wakefield was not available I saw someone else in his surgery when I went with a minor health problem. I had not spoken about the abuse for about 3 years apart from to my second husband. It was time to try again because I realized that I needed help. I didn't want to risk this marriage breaking up because I was an unfeeling partner during love-making. I don't think the GP even heard what I was telling him. He never even looked up from writing a prescription. He didn't say a word. I had learned by then if I ever wanted to tell someone about the abuse I had to put all those years, all the pain and all the effects the abuse had on me, into two or three sentences because I never had more time to talk about it. I was always interrupted with some patronizing remark. This time I didn't wait to recover from being rejected in my need for help. Within days I saw a female doctor in the family planning clinic and told her the same story. Her advice to overcome my dislike of physical contact was to 'satisfy myself' or to 'use a vibrator', if I couldn't find pleasure with a man. To a victim of sexual abuse who looks on sex as dirty and degrading this is the most unhelpful suggestion possible.

Every time I told someone the emptiness in me grew. I was so eager to find some response, someone saying 'Tell me about it, I'll help you'. I knew what my brother did was wrong, I wanted reassurance that it was wrong, someone reinforcing my belief that it was his fault that I wasn't feeling the way other women feel.

I tried to talk about it a few more times to people, mostly friends. They hardly acknowledged what they heard, none of them was supportive. Then I gave up. I resigned myself to never being able to enjoy sex; always having thoughts that I was less worthy than others; never losing the fear that my son would abuse his sisters; and all the other problems that I knew resulted from the sexual abuse I suffered as a child.

Suddenly I had some personal tragedies which had nothing to do with my past. They came within a few weeks of each other and I became depressed. After 3 weeks I went to see one of the GPs in my surgery. I told her about my depression, expecting to get some drugs to help. I gave her all the reasons why I thought things were getting too much for me. Again I mentioned in two sentences that I was abused as a child. For the first time in my life someone looked at me with sympathy, encouraging me to carry on talking about it. We talked for about 10 minutes and never before was I allowed to say so much about how I felt it had affected me all my life. She told me about the survivors' groups and asked if I would be interested in joining them. I almost cried with relief. Yes, I was interested.

The new group had just started so I had to wait 3 months before I could join but from that day onwards I felt protected. I saw that even though over 30 years had passed since I first looked for help, it was not too late. We can change our lives no matter how long it takes. The hardest part for me was always the moments just after telling someone, when I was not believed or told to forget it. But whenever I felt close to giving up I thought that somewhere, someone must care. I just had to find that person. Now I think that perseverance was the right way for me. If I had given up trying, I would not be the woman I am now. I am happier now and more fulfilled than I have ever been before. **Ingrid**

Perhaps each of us can also be ready to listen and believe if someone (male or female, child or adult) chooses to disclose sexual abuse to us.

Exercises

1 If you have had a bad response when you've talked about your sexual abuse, try writing down what happened and why you think the person responded in this way. Remember the problem is within them, not you.
2 Think about talking to someone about what has happened to you. Look at 'Sources of help' at the back of this book. It gives suggestions about who you can tell and how to get help. If you phone one of the helplines, you will be listened to, and you will be believed. If you don't get an appropriate response, find someone else to talk to.
3 If you want to know how to respond if a child or an adult discloses sexual abuse to you, or if you suspect abuse, see Chapter 16 on 'Working towards prevention'.

Part 3
TACKLING THE PROBLEMS

7

Buried feelings

The ability to experience and express many different emotions – happiness, sadness, anger, grief, love, hate, fear and joy – is a natural part of being human. Sometimes, however, feelings are too intense, overwhelming or painful to be experienced or expressed directly. Some of the difficulties that survivors have in adult life are caused by the ways they have learnt to cope with their painful thoughts and feelings about the abuse, both as children and as adults. The capacity to 'cut off' from bad experiences, whether conscious or unconscious, protects abused children and young people from fully experiencing the horror of the situation they are in. After the sexual abuse has ended, survivors may consciously try to forget about it and find ways to push their memories and feelings away (avoidance); or they may unconsciously cut off altogether so they have no feelings about the event or are unable to remember what happened (dissociation). Avoidance and dissociation are described below.

Avoidance – burying feelings and memories

Abused children and young people often hide their anger and distress from other people so that no one will suspect they are being abused. They may also keep their feelings rigidly under control while they are being abused to try to protect themselves from their distress and pain, or because they do not want the abuser to see how much he or she is hurting them. After the abuse has stopped, adult survivors may continue to cope by trying to push their feelings away and trying to forget that the abuse ever happened. However, the feelings and memories that people try to bury usually surface at times in some form, and cause either physical or emotional problems and distress. Facing memories and feelings can be painful, but by finding new ways to express and process your memories and feelings, instead of blocking them off, you can begin to heal.

Survivors often learn to cope with difficult emotions or memories by using avoidance – for example, by consciously blocking memories and feelings, and in time this can become an automatic process. Some of the ways people avoid experiencing their feelings, and the kinds of problems this can cause, are described below.

AVOIDING TRIGGERS

Survivors often find ways to avoid thinking about their childhood abuse, or to avoid their feelings about what has happened. They may keep themselves busy and distracted, or make sure they are never alone, so they don't have time to think. Some survivors do the same thing again and again when their memories and feelings begin to surface – for example, washing themselves, cleaning, counting or checking things.

Survivors often try to avoid any triggers that might remind them of the abuse and cause their feelings and memories to surface. They may particularly avoid anything to do with sex or sexual abuse (in television programmes, conversations, books, the internet) or anything that reminds them of their childhood (photographs, people, places, children).

> Some years ago, I got out all my childhood photos. My brother was on many of them. I tore up the parts of the photos with his image and destroyed everything that reminded me of him. Yet the memories remained. **Katarina**

Some survivors avoid people who are expressing strong emotions – for example, other people crying or shouting, because they fear it will bring up their own feelings. They may or may not be aware of what they are doing. Some survivors describe mentally locking away their memories and feelings in a secure box.

Survivors are often encouraged to behave like this by friends or advisers, who say that the best thing they can do is put the abuse behind them and get on with their lives. However, the memories and feelings do not go away; they are still there. For a time, they may be less accessible and less troublesome, but this method of coping can lead to other problems.

Avoiding memories and feelings by keeping busy, finding distractions or repeatedly counting, checking or cleaning can be very stressful and lead to high levels of anxiety, phobias and obsessions.

I was unable to express my feelings due to the constant battle to hide my secret and contain my fears. I perpetually felt like I was bottling up my feelings and would explode. I wouldn't let anyone near me. I always played the joker or the agony aunt – I talked to other people about them not me. I was always trying to look normal. I also became obsessional about working out. **Luke**

I pushed the memories and feelings away by cleaning excessively, brushing my teeth ten times and more a day, banging my head, slashing my wrists and burning myself. **Graham**

Adult survivors often become so expert at cutting off from distressing feelings that they do this automatically.

No matter what bad thing happened in my life, I could not cry. I could not feel any emotions. For most years of my adult life, I was emotionally dead. I was neither happy nor sad, neither depressed nor angry. I simply felt nothing. Even when I was almost daily abused during my first marriage it did not cause me the pain it should have done. Most of the time it did not bother me. I was too frightened to accept feelings of any kind. **Ingrid**

At first I used to have to concentrate and force myself to push the feelings and memories away. I blocked them over with different thoughts. Now it just happens without any effort – it's automatic. I even managed to forget about the abuse totally for 12 years. **Rhys**

Fiona had learnt to avoid her feelings about being abused and later realized that she had cut off from all kinds of bad feelings.

When I was talking to my daughter about growing up I started telling her about when I was 17 and my mum left home. Something suddenly hit me. I had never really noticed that my mum had left my life. It was as if I didn't care. I must have been so hardened to pain or pushed my emotions so deeply away that I couldn't feel the full extent of the hurt. Looking back now I get the stab of emotions, the emptiness, the betrayal. My sadness now as a mother myself could be the scars I bear from the kind of emotional upsets I suffered growing up.

I never really grieved about a lot of things, like the death of my grandad. I missed my grandad. I couldn't stand the emptiness I felt inside. I often wanted to cry but most times I wouldn't let myself. Even today I do the same. I feel ashamed to cry. I feel I'm attention-seeking and feeling sorry for myself so I get angry with myself and afraid about what people will think. **Fiona**

PHYSICAL TENSION

Feelings and memories can be held back by physical tension. Children learn at an early age to hold back tears by tensing their chest and face muscles. Anger, grief and rage can also be held in by tensing any part of the body. We talk about people becoming 'rigid with rage' or 'bowed down with grief'. These figures of speech convey very vividly how unexpressed feelings can affect the physical body.

It requires a great deal of physical tension and mental energy to hold back feelings and memories. Tensing the body can also become an automatic response. It saps energy and can lead to chronic tension, headaches, aches and pains and many other physical symptoms. It also keeps the body in a heightened state of stress and makes people more vulnerable to anxiety, panic attacks, illness and injury.

FOOD, ALCOHOL AND DRUGS

Food, alcohol and drugs can be used as ways of blocking off bad feelings. Eating food can bring immediate comfort and enable people to distract themselves from their difficult emotions and eventually block them out completely. Alcohol and drugs (both legal and illegal) work in a similar way by allowing people to block out the pain and cut off from reality.

Alcohol, drugs and food can seem very attractive ways of dealing with distressing feelings, memories and situations, because they are easy to take and quick to work, but they are only short-term ways of blocking out distress. Using alcohol, drugs and food to cope on a regular basis can bring their own problems and so create serious difficulties.

> I blocked out my feelings by drinking alcohol excessively. I used alcohol as an escape from my thoughts, although this was only a temporary measure. I got myself into trouble with the police due to the amount of alcohol I was consuming. I was aggressive at times, had mood swings and got arrested for being drunk and disorderly. **Anthony**

PASSING OUT
Some survivors pass out, or black out, when there is no physical reason for this to occur. This may have happened to them first as a child during the abuse. Blackouts can happen to adult survivors because something triggers bad memories and feelings about the abuse. By passing out, they enter a state in which they can no longer consciously think or feel. When they come round, they may have no memory of what caused them to pass out.

Blackouts can be frightening experiences, and falling down without any warning is physically dangerous. Lucy passed out when anything reminded her of the abuse or her abuser. She was briefly protected from her emotional pain, but her blackouts became more and more frequent, and she often injured herself when she fell down. Eventually, she was unable to work or lead a normal life and was referred to a neurologist. When the neurologist found nothing physically wrong with her, she was referred to the psychology service. As she began to deal with the consequences of her childhood abuse, her blackouts became less frequent and eventually stopped.

OTHER WAYS OF AVOIDING
In addition to the methods mentioned above, some survivors push away their memories and feelings by compulsively caring for other people, by sleeping all the time, with excessive exercise or by harming themselves.

Many of the above coping strategies begin as deliberate ways for people to try to take control of their own emotions, but they can easily become automatic responses. Survivors then respond to triggers by shutting down their emotions, or consuming a substance to 'swallow' their feelings, without any forethought; and in doing so, they lose any control over the process. All these coping strategies that block off memories and feelings can develop into problems in themselves.

Dissociation

Dissociating, or 'cutting off', is another way in which people can survive dreadful experiences by escaping from their painful thoughts and feelings. It is normal for all children to dissociate. They may get totally immersed in a television programme or a game; have an imaginary friend; or drift off into a fantasy world in lessons at school. As children grow up, they generally tend to dissociate less and less, although most adults will still dissociate in threatening situations.

When children are being sexually abused, they often dissociate, or separate off, from their bodies, so that they do not feel the physical or emotional pain. Some children describe stepping outside their bodies and watching themselves being abused, without experiencing any of the pain. They describe it as if it is another child experiencing the abuse and they are merely observers. Others invent a fantasy world into which they can retreat every time they are being abused, so they are not mentally present or fully aware during the abuse and may have little or no memory of it afterwards. Some survivors dissociate by distancing themselves from the traumatic experience; others protect themselves by putting the difficult experience into a locked box or a compartment. Dissociating is an automatic process that can protect children from extreme or confusing situations, and some children and young people learn to dissociate whenever they feel under threat.

Dissociating is a common way in which children cope with the horror of being sexually abused. Children who have survived being abused in this way tend to continue to dissociate in particular situations as they grow up. Adult survivors tend to dissociate whenever thoughts or feelings about the abuse are triggered; this cuts them off and protects them from the painful memories. This can happen automatically in situations where the adults feel they cannot cope or feel overwhelmed by their emotions. Afterwards, the survivor may feel confused and not understand what has happened.

Dissociating may initially happen at times when the survivor is feeling overwhelmed, but, as mentioned above, it can develop into an automatic response to a wider range of situations. This early coping strategy can then become a serious problem where the survivors feel they are losing control of their lives. Adult survivors sometimes go into a dissociated state for hours or days at a time. When they come out of this state, they are often confused about what they have been doing, or how they got to be where they are. They have sometimes been going about their everyday tasks but may have appeared a little vague or different from usual. People in dissociated states may appear to be drunk or on drugs.

Survivors who dissociate from physical pain as children may find that they do not feel pain as adults; for example, they may be able to have dental procedures without an anaesthetic. 'Passing out', as described above, could be another form of dissociation. Some survivors 'lose' time or find they have said and done things which they have no memory of. Dissociating can be a very frightening experience. Survivors may feel they are going mad or that there is something seriously physically wrong with them. Many are sent to see neurologists or to have other physical examinations.

SPLITTING INTO SEPARATE PARTS

All forms of sexual abuse can have a damaging impact, but some children experience particularly severe and prolonged abuse, where, for example, there is no hope of escape, no one to protect or comfort the child *and* the sexual acts are extreme, and there is physical violence, confinement or terrifying threats. If sexual abuse begins when the child is very young, and the abuse is very severe, children have to find drastic ways to survive the overwhelming terror and helplessness. The severely abused child can be so over-whelmed by the terror, shame or extreme acts involved in the abuse that they have to split off from it, or dissociate.

We all have different parts of our personality that come through at different times – for example, people often say they feel and act differently as soon as they put their work clothes or uniform on, and some people act very differently from usual when they are driving a car. The overwhelming emotions or the horrific experiences of abuse may be held in one of the parts of the child's personality, but in extreme situations this part becomes split off from the child's awareness in order to protect the child. In this situation, once this process begins, other overwhelming events or emotions may also be split off, resulting in several walled-off parts of the child's personality. These parts or identities help the children survive the overwhelming feelings and experiences of the abuse by carrying, or containing, the split-off traumatic events and emotions.

If children have to dissociate like this for a prolonged period, walls or barriers are likely to be developed between the different parts to hold the terrible experiences at bay and out of the child's awareness. This can result in the survivor having different parts or identities that may control their thoughts and behaviour at different times. These different identities or parts of the survivor may not know that the other parts exist, or they may think the other parts are separate people with different bodies.

Survivors who have developed different, separate, parts of themselves may discover that they feel and behave very differently at different times; and sometimes do and say things that seem completely out of character. They may also have big gaps in their memory. This extreme form of dissociation comes into operation to help the young child survive overwhelming and extreme abuse where there is no hope of escape, and is called dissociative identity disorder or multiple personality disorder. If you think you may have dissociative identity disorder, seek help from your GP or another source or visit the Positive Outcomes for Dissociative Survivors (PODS) website for information about dissociative disorders and support (see 'Sources of help').

Memories and feelings surface

Survivors cannot be sure of being able to hold back memories and feelings if the underlying cause, the sexual abuse, is not dealt with. Memories and emotions may come back through dreams and flashbacks, or surface unexpectedly. Feelings about the abuse can sometimes be transferred on to other people and situations; for example, you may get angry at your boss because he reminds you of your abuser. Dreams are a way in which hidden memories and feelings can come back into consciousness, and can be useful ways of processing bad experiences.

Survivors sometimes have nightmares relating to the abuse. These nightmares are usually not directly about the abuse but relate to survivors' feelings and memories about it – for example, nightmares about survivors' childhood, the abuser, death, sex, being in danger and being chased or trapped. Nightmares are discussed in Chapter 8, 'Anxiety, fears and trauma'.

Flashbacks are another way in which blocked memories and feelings can surface. When a person has a flashback, it feels as if they are vividly re-experiencing past traumatic events. During a flashback, the survivor may feel like he or she is a child again and is reliving the abuse. Flashbacks can happen at any time; the survivor has no conscious control over them. They can be triggered by reminders of the abuse and therefore often occur during sex. Like all forms of memory, flashbacks and nightmares are open to distortion and may not accurately represent past events.

Many things can remind survivors of their abuse, and they may not always be able to avoid the triggers. Survivors who try to push away their memories, or have dissociated from them, are vulnerable to being suddenly reminded of the abuse and may find themselves taken unawares by memories flooding back. This can happen in situations where it is very difficult to deal with them; Dorothy's memories came flooding back when she went into labour.

Painful feelings can also come rushing back. Fits of rage, or floods of tears for no apparent reason, are frequently described by survivors. Survivors may be taken by surprise by their emotions and be unable to understand where they are coming from and what they are about. Many women believe they are at the mercy of their hormones, suffering from premenstrual tension, postnatal depression, the menopause or some chemical imbalance. Survivors may be treated for these problems, or for anxiety and depression, for many years without making the link between their overpowering emotions and the past sexual abuse.

Feelings can also surface and be transferred on to other people or other situations where they can be more easily expressed. Survivors who feel very little about their own abuse may find themselves weeping profusely at a film or book, or mad with rage at an injustice that has been done to another person. They may find themselves getting angry at people for trivial reasons.

> I was angry but I didn't know what at and so it was vented at my husband, the dog, anyone close to me. **Jocelyn**

Difficulties in relationships and sexual problems can also be the result of unresolved feelings about the abuse or abuser. The survivor's buried feelings about the abuse surface and are transferred on to a current relationship.

Facing buried feelings – when and why?

As we have seen, many mental health problems such as anxiety, depression, phobias, sexual problems, eating disorders, drug addiction and tension can be the result of unprocessed feelings and memories from being sexually abused. A history of sexual abuse is frequently linked to a wide range of psychiatric disorders. Survivors have often received many years of treatment for these surface problems before the underlying problem of the sexual abuse is uncovered and dealt with.

Survivors eventually come to a point where the old coping strategies that push the abuse away are no longer working, or are becoming serious problems in themselves. Feelings and memories may be surfacing despite attempts to bury them, or flashbacks may be triggered during everyday activities. At this point, survivors may decide that they have to get help and that they need to disclose the abuse. They may have carried their secret for 10, 20, even 50 years before this happens. In some cases, specific events cause memories and feelings about the abuse to surface.

> Last year I had a little girl who only lived an hour and then died. I thought I'd coped with it quite well but my mother had been no help whatsoever – she only came to see me once. I felt as though she'd let me down – everything accentuated how I'd felt for a long time about myself. I didn't like myself at all. I was really depressed and one day I told my health visitor that I'd been sexually abused as a child. I hadn't thought about it a lot but then I realized that was my problem. The death of my little girl brought back that my mother wasn't there for me, all those years ago, she didn't protect me then either. That's what triggered off my depression. **Jocelyn**

Jocelyn had been abused by two men 22 years earlier. She had struggled with her feelings and memories all those years by trying to push them away; but the death of her baby, and the lack of response from her mother, meant she was no longer able to keep them at bay. This prompted her to disclose her sexual abuse and then get help by joining a survivors' group.

> I don't think I could have gone for help before. There's a point when it's right to go – for me it was my mum letting me down again and I could see it this time. Before, although I felt so bad, I didn't realize I needed help or that anything could help. **Jocelyn**

Rhys's feelings and memories also surfaced because of events in his life.

I got a back injury playing rugby. I was laid up and couldn't get to my son's birth. I got depressed. More and more memories came up and I was flooded with emotion. That's when my GP recommended that I get help. **Rhys**

Sometimes survivors seek help because of the effect the abuse is having on their relationship:

I went for help because I became aggressive and I could not go on shouting and snapping at my wife. **Graham**

Getting into a relationship may also mean the abuse begins to surface.

I fell in love with an individual who refused to let me stay insular and demanded to know everything about me. Once I began telling, the pressure became intense and I felt close to a nervous breakdown so I sought help. **Luke**

Some survivors may have to reach a stage where they feel absolutely desperate, or attempt to end their life, before they start to talk about the abuse.

I was getting suicidal. I felt I was totally losing control and that I didn't have the right to make decisions. I always used to feel in control at work but now this was starting to crumble as well as everything else. I went to see my GP for a referral to clinical psychology. **Jane**

Anthony's use of alcohol led to increasing problems with the police. Luckily, his need for help was eventually recognized.

I had been put on probation so many times the courts didn't know what to do with me. Then I told them about my abuse and my probation officer got help for me. **Anthony**

Lucy had blacked out whenever her memories and feelings about the abuse were triggered, but when this started to become a serious problem, she decided to get help.

I kept having blackouts and being admitted to hospital. They couldn't find anything physically wrong with me and so referred me to a psychologist. I was so desperate that I either had to do something and get it right or kill myself. I decided it was time I really got to the bottom of it. **Lucy**

Like Lucy, some survivors eventually get psychological help after they have been through a wide range of medical tests and investigations. Their physical symptoms (blackouts, fits, numbness, pains, gynaecological problems) are sometimes found to be a result of the trauma of childhood sexual abuse.

> I never used to cry or even get upset, I'd always black out. During one survivor's group meeting, however, I burst into tears. Crying made me feel better and I felt as if I could talk about the abuse. Feelings of anger also came out in the group. Before I was always 'fine' and didn't need help but I kept having blackouts and I think I would have killed myself if I hadn't got help. Now I can say 'I'm not all right' and I don't have to put a brave face on it.
> Lucy

Some of the problems that result from burying feelings are discussed in more detail in the following chapters. We discuss ways of managing the problems, but to overcome them you also need to find ways to express and process the underlying feelings and memories about the sexual abuse. When powerful feelings and memories begin to surface, it can be frightening and disturbing. However, it does mean that they can now be experienced and dealt with, even if the abuse happened many years ago. Allowing your buried feelings and memories to surface is the first step. Being truly in touch with your feelings not only helps to heal the past, but also allows you to experience life more fully and openly in the present.

Exercises and suggestions

1 Write a list of any ways in which you have tried to block or push away your memories and feelings – for example, avoiding (places, people, thoughts); keeping busy; distracting yourself; obsessively doing something (counting, checking, cleaning); using alcohol, drugs or food; sleeping; excessive exercise. It may be that the process of pushing away your bad feelings is automatic, rather than deliberate, as with dissociating or passing out.

2 Look at Box 5 below, and tick off any events that have triggered your memories and feelings about the abuse.

3 Look at the symptoms of PTSD in Box 2 in Chapter 2. If you are dissociating, or struggling to cope with symptoms such as flashbacks, you are probably suffering from the effects of unpro-

---

Box 5 Events that trigger memories and feelings about child sexual abuse

Below are some of the events and situations that may reawaken buried memories and feelings about the abuse.

- Birth of a baby girl.
- Birth of a baby boy.
- Child reaching the age when the survivor's abuse started.
- Death of the abuser.
- Death of a non-abusing parent of the survivor.
- Meeting or seeing a person who looks like the abuser.
- Revisiting the place of the abuse.
- Hearing or reading about another person's abuse.
- Feeling vulnerable, ill or under stress.
- Any situation in which a survivor once again feels:
  - stigmatized, such as if falsely accused of stealing;
  - betrayed, such as partner having an affair;
  - powerless, such as losing his or her job;
  - sexually traumatized, such as rape, revenge porn.

---

cessed trauma, or possibly PTSD. It is very difficult to deal with these symptoms on your own. Please think about getting some help for yourself (EMDR therapy or trauma-focused CBT) – see 'Sources of help', which also includes the PODS website for information about dissociative disorders.

4 Some survivors are overwhelmed by their feelings, but others have lost touch with their emotions. If you are out of touch with how you feel and want to make contact with your feelings again, do the following exercise. During the next few days, keep pausing and ask yourself 'What am I feeling now?', and notice what is happening in your body. Do this regularly every day and make a note of your feelings. Put a coloured piece of sticky paper on your watch or phone (or on something else you look at regularly) to remind you to notice your feelings every time you look at it.

5 The chapters on 'Coping strategies' and 'Dealing with emotions, flashbacks and hallucinations' in the *Breaking Free Workbook* may be useful in helping you manage triggers and cope with strong emotions and surfacing memories.

8

Anxiety, fears and trauma

Not being able to eat in front of people came on gradually – it just seemed to get worse and worse. It was as if everybody was watching me. **Mavis**

When I had my first panic attack I didn't know what was happening. I just felt a fear that I had never experienced before. I was scared to tell anyone because I thought I was cracking up and they would think I was really stupid. **Polly**

Many survivors of childhood sexual abuse feel tense and nervous much of the time. Others can't stop worrying all the time. Some survivors cannot travel alone, avoid busy shops, are unable to eat in front of people, have panic attacks or think everybody is looking at them. Other survivors have intense fears of specific things, like being in the dark or older men. Many have experienced so much fear as children and young people that, as adults, their minds and bodies are still alert and constantly looking out for danger. These are all symptoms of anxiety, and while many people suffer with anxiety, it is particularly common in those who have suffered abuse in childhood. Some survivors have been traumatized by the events of their childhood and have lasting symptoms of trauma, including nightmares, hallucinations and flashbacks, and may even have PTSD.

In this chapter, we look at the range of symptoms and problems experienced by people who suffer from anxiety or one of the anxiety disorders, as well as providing ideas to help you reduce and manage these symptoms. We then discuss some of the symptoms resulting from being involved in a traumatic event, such as sexual abuse, with suggestions of the best ways to manage or resolve them.

Anxiety

Experiencing anxiety is normal for everyone, and most people feel anxious at times – for example, when attending a job interview, going somewhere they have not been before or meeting new people. The symptoms of anxiety can be mild or severe; they may only last until a stressful event is over, or the person may continue to feel anxious for many years. Feeling anxious develops from being a normal part of life into a problem or disorder when people feel anxious a lot of the time, the symptoms are interfering with their lives, or they can no longer control their symptoms and feel like the anxiety is in control of them.

When people feel anxious, their minds and bodies are in a state of fear even when they are not in actual danger. They may say they are feeling scared, nervous, afraid, anxious or worried. People with high levels of anxiety are usually very tense and may describe themselves as 'jumpy', 'nervy' or 'wound-up'. Some people worry all the time about anything and everything (generalized anxiety disorder); others have specific fears and phobias; many have panic attacks; some check, count or clean all the time (obsessive compulsive disorder – OCD); and some people develop complex phobias such as agoraphobia and social phobia.

SYMPTOMS OF ANXIETY

People who have problems with anxiety experience a wide range of symptoms that can be grouped as follows: physical symptoms, changes in behaviour and negative thoughts. Box 6 contains a list of the more common symptoms of anxiety; have a look and see how many apply to you. Understanding these are just symptoms of anxiety, rather than that there is something wrong with you or that you have lost control over what is happening to you, can help you work on reducing your symptoms and get back in control of your life.

Box 6 Common symptoms of anxiety

Physical symptoms include:
- tension
- palpitations (becoming aware of your heartbeat)
- 'butterflies' in the stomach

- trembling, shaking
- pins and needles
- feeling short of breath
- loss of appetite
- poor sleep
- sweating
- chest pain
- dry mouth
- weak legs
- aches and pains
- vomiting
- diarrhoea
- blurred vision
- surroundings seeming unreal
- nausea
- poor concentration
- dizziness
- churning stomach
- headache.

Common behaviours include:
- drinking too much
- eating too much
- eating too little
- taking drugs (prescribed or illegal)
- avoiding going to places
- escaping from places where you feel afraid
- obsessional cleaning, counting or checking
- keeping busy
- worrying about anything.

Negative thoughts include:
- 'I'm going to have a heart attack.'
- 'Everyone can tell what I'm really like.'
- 'My children are going to have a bad accident.'
- 'I'm cracking up. I'm going to end up in the mental hospital.'
- 'Everyone is talking about me.'
- 'I will lose control/go crazy.'
- 'I'm going to faint or pass out.'
- 'I will not be able to breathe.'
- 'I can't cope with anything.'
- 'People think I'm dirty.'

PHYSICAL SYMPTOMS

When people are anxious, they experience the same physical reactions as people do when they are in actual danger. When people are in danger, their bodies increase the production of stress hormones (adrenaline and cortisol). This is known as the 'flight-or-fight' response, which helps people deal with dangerous situations by preparing the body for action.

People who are anxious, however, experience these bodily symptoms even when they are not in danger. Many of the physical symptoms of anxiety, such as palpitations, butterflies in the stomach and dry mouth, are caused by the body's natural response to danger. People often begin to breathe quickly or gasp for air (hyperventilation) when they are afraid. This rapid breathing causes changes in the chemistry of the blood, creating physical changes associated with anxiety (such as shortness of breath, pins and needles, and dizziness). People also tense their muscles in response to fear, and this can develop into a habit, resulting in aches and pains in many parts of the body.

NEGATIVE THOUGHTS

When people are anxious, they may worry all the time or have recurrent negative thoughts about themselves or others. They often assume that something dreadful is going to happen – for example, 'I'll never see my children again.' Anxious people can have negative thoughts about benign events. They may, for example, notice somebody looking at them ('being looked at' is a trigger for them) and think, 'Everyone is looking at me, they can see what I'm really like.' The negative thoughts may be connected to the physical symptoms of anxiety, as they are in the examples given below:

Physical symptoms	Negative thoughts
Feeling dizzy.	'I'm going to pass out.'
Tingling sensation.	'I'm having a stroke.'
Blurred vision, things look unreal.	'I'm going mad – I'll end up in the mental hospital.'

This kind of thinking is called catastrophizing, in this case making a catastrophe out of the harmless (but uncomfortable) physical symptoms of fear. Negative thoughts make anxiety symptoms worse, which then increases feelings of anxiety. This rise in anxiety produces more of the physical symptoms and starts a vicious circle of increasing fear.

BEHAVIOURAL CHANGES
When people feel anxious, they often change their behaviour to try to cope with how they are feeling. If they feel very anxious in a particular situation, they may have a strong urge to escape, and sometimes they do run away. If they leave the situation, they do not discover that the catastrophe they believe will happen (for example, they will faint or be humiliated) does not happen. They may feel embarrassed that people saw them run out, and this may make it harder for them to return to that situation. People sometimes start to avoid places where they have been afraid because they fear they will become anxious there again. If you avoid situations where you have previously been afraid, you lose the opportunity to learn that it is not the situation that is dangerous – it is how you react in that situation that triggers your anxiety and fear.

Other common ways of coping with feelings of anxiety include eating more, taking tablets or drinking alcohol. These behaviours may reduce the fear for a short time, but trying to avoid fear by using any of these coping strategies actually increases the fear in the long term. Unfortunately, all these ways of trying to cope with anxiety can become habits and, in time, develop into problems themselves such as agoraphobia, binge-eating, dependence on medication, alcohol abuse and obsessional behaviour.

LINKS WITH SEXUAL ABUSE
It is normal for anyone to be anxious in worrying or threatening situations. When people are chronically anxious, they have often experienced a great deal of fear, or have been in a dangerous or threatening situation, for a period of time. Their bodies continue to respond with symptoms of fear in everyday situations, even when they are no longer in actual danger. Children and young people who are being abused may feel fearful or terrified for much of their childhood: afraid they will be sexually abused again; afraid the abuser will do something worse; afraid they are being physically damaged by the abuse; afraid they will get pregnant; afraid that people can tell they are being abused; or afraid of the consequences if anyone finds out. Their sense of safety has been shattered, and

it is difficult for them to relax and feel secure; they are always on alert for danger.

When children and young people experience fear like this for long stretches of time, it is unlikely that this fear will just disappear when the abuse stops or they become adults. They have learnt to be fearful and will probably continue to experience the symptoms of fear until they understand *why* they are anxious, learn how to control their symptoms and work on the fear, guilt and other issues resulting from the abuse.

Panic attacks

Panic attacks are an extreme form of anxiety, usually triggered by thoughts and memories. They are very frightening because the physical symptoms are powerful and unexpected. People often think they are about to experience something catastrophic – for example, they are going to have a heart attack, suffocate, lose control, go 'crazy' or even die. These negative thoughts make people even more frightened and so increase the physical symptoms and the tension. This in turn leads to more negative thoughts and causes the panic to build up and up.

When people have panic attacks, they experience a very strong urge to run away, and may actually do so. Running away from the situation may make them feel relieved, briefly, but will make the fear worse in the long run. People who suffer with anxiety are usually afraid something bad is going to happen in the future; during a panic attack, it feels like the bad thing is going to happen *right now*.

Survivors may have intense and sudden attacks of anxiety when they think about their abuse or are in situations associated with their abuse.

> The first time that I can remember having a panic attack was when I was about 10 years old. I was at a Christmas party at my grandma's house. Three of my abusers were present at the party. I remember feeling very frightened and very dizzy. My heart was thumping very hard, I could feel all the pulses in my body going and I started shaking all over. I felt very faint and weak. At the time I didn't realize what was happening. I didn't realize I was having a panic attack. **Wendy**

Some survivors, like Wendy, started having panic attacks as children, but many develop them for the first time as adults.

> At the time of my first panic attack, I was having flashbacks and nightmares about the sexual abuse by my grandfather. I tried to push the memories down and get on with my everyday life but the panic attacks kept happening. **Polly**

Taking control of panic attacks

Appendix 1 describes how to breathe properly, provides more information about panic attacks and explains how you can gain control of them.

Please read Appendix 1 now if you haven't already, practise breathing properly and learn how to manage panic attacks. It is possible to manage panic attacks and become more in control of your fear and anxiety in your day-to-day life.

Fears and phobias

Some survivors are not only generally anxious, but also suffer from specific fears. These fears can develop into phobias – irrational and sometimes overwhelming fears of specific things or situations.

> I'm frightened to death of spiders and can't go upstairs if there is one around. **Rhys**

People can develop phobias associated with situations where they have had traumatic experiences; for example, people who have been involved in a car crash may become phobic about travelling in cars; or a child who is bitten by a dog may grow into an adult who is phobic about dogs. Some people, though, are not aware of how their specific fear began. People often develop phobias about situations (being in a supermarket, in a group of people, near a particular animal, in the dark) where they have felt anxious or had panic attacks. The initial fear can develop into a phobia if the person continually avoids getting into that situation again; this allows the fear of that situation to grow. The person's lifestyle becomes restricted as they avoid more and more situations. In this section, we describe some of the fears and phobias that are most commonly associated with sexual abuse: specific phobias, more complex phobias such as agoraphobia and social phobia, and obsessional/compulsive problems.

FEARS ASSOCIATED WITH THE ABUSER

Survivors often have fears that are associated with the person, or people, who abused them: fears of body hair; the smell of alcohol; cigarette smoke; being kissed by older men; specific clothing, uniforms or hairstyles; particular perfumes or smells; men generally. As adults, both male and female survivors who have been abused by men may be frightened of all men or of a specific group of men – for example, older men, men with beards or men who smell of alcohol. Kate was abused by several men and as an adult was frightened of being alone with a man.

> When I went into a shop I hated men serving me. Sometimes I wouldn't go into a shop at all unless I thought a woman would serve me. **Kate**

Some abusers seem to go into a semi-trance while they are abusing (the abuser may be dissociating). Survivors often describe the glazed look in the eyes of their abusers before or during the abuse and, as adults, become fearful if they see someone with eyes that look glazed over.

FEARS ASSOCIATED WITH THE ABUSE

Some fears and phobias develop because of their association with the situation where the survivor was abused or with objects used during the abuse. Survivors often have fears of bathrooms, being in a room with a closed door, the dark, being touched, washing their hair or being alone at night. Abuse often occurs in the dark or behind closed doors. Many children are abused in bathrooms; abusers who are family members often take advantage of a child taking a bath or washing their hair, and use this as an opportunity to abuse them. As a young adult, Graham was raped in a public toilet by three men. He now has a fear of using public toilets as well as a fear of being among men. Survivors develop fears of being touched in certain ways, on certain parts of the body or by particular people; these fears are usually associated with the touching they experienced during the abuse.

Survivors may also have fears relating to objects used during the abuse: knives used to threaten the child, bottles or other objects that were inserted into the child's anus or vagina. Lucy passed out whenever ice cream was mentioned; her abuser had smeared her with ice cream.

Claustrophobia (the fear of being in an enclosed space) can also develop from being locked in a room or cupboard, or from feeling trapped during the abuse. Adult fears, which may seem to be irrational, can often be traced back to an association with the abuser, the situation the abuse occurred in, or the threats that accompanied the abuse; and these fears can be triggered by everyday events.

SPECIFIC FEARS AND MEDICAL APPOINTMENTS
Some of the specific fears associated with the abuse, as described above, can result in fear and difficulty when medical or dental examinations and procedures are required. You may be avoiding medical or dental examinations because of specific fears such as being afraid of being touched, of having objects inserted into your body, of being trapped or confined or of medical professionals. This may be putting your health, or even your life, at risk, and it is another way the past abuse is continuing to harm you.

Try to find out what it is in the medical or dental situation that triggers your fear and practise the breathing exercises given in Appendix 1 – or whatever self-calming technique works for you – while imagining the trigger situation; keep repeating this until you feel less afraid. Tell your doctor, nurse or dentist that you have difficulty in that situation (you do not have to give the reason why, unless you want to, many people are terrified of dentistry and medical appointments). Talk to the professionals involved about what will help you cope in the situation (for example, taking it slowly, stopping whenever you signal, taking a friend in with you). Some survivors avoid medical procedures because they are scared they will be terrified by a hallucination of their abuser (that is, they may see the abuser in the room threatening them when the abuser is not really there). If this applies to you, read about trauma-based hallucinations and how to manage them later on in this chapter.

If you cannot manage to attend for examinations using these suggestions, please seek help. Don't let the abuser continue to put your health at risk.

AGORAPHOBIA

The first panic attack I put down to being tired and under stress but they kept happening to me. They made me so frightened that I was scared to go out or do anything for fear of having one. If I went out I would start feeling really shaky and my heart would be thumping. I would sweat and I felt dizzy like I was going to pass out. I had to leave wherever I was. I just needed to run and get away, preferably home where it would go away. I gave up work and became like a hermit. My friends and relatives all tried to help but I wouldn't admit to them what was happening to me. I made excuses: too tired, headache, felt sick – anything to get out of going out. I tried going back to work but I was really nervous. I seemed to cope for a while and then again from nowhere I had another panic. I stopped work and became really depressed, thinking I was cracking up and would end up locked up in a nut house. **Polly**

Some survivors of sexual abuse, like Polly, develop agoraphobia – an intense fear of being away from the perceived safety of the home, being in busy places or feeling trapped. People who suffer from agoraphobia often fear travelling on public transport, standing in a queue, being in a busy place, being alone or being out of the house.

I hate crowded places such as supermarkets and shopping malls. Sometimes I try to overcome this but it is not easy for me. **Anthony**

Sometimes on a bus I feel like everyone is staring at me. I want to run and hide – I feel threatened. **Rhys**

Some people with agoraphobia feel safe enough to go outside if they are in or near their car, or if they have someone else with them. They may feel threatened and anxious when they are outside their own homes and develop a fear of leaving the house. Survivors have often felt trapped and out of control during the abuse, and these feelings can return whenever they are in situations that they cannot immediately leave, such as waiting at supermarket checkouts.

Fear and panic die down in time by themselves, but if you leave the situation, you do not learn that your fear would have died down anyway. You begin to believe that you are afraid of the situation itself, when actually it is your negative thoughts in that situation that trigger the fear. When you go into that situation again, you are more likely to want to leave because you escaped last time and felt better. This may happen in more and more places until eventually there are few places where you feel comfortable. Fears experienced during the abuse, such as being trapped or feeling out of control, can develop into a more general fear of the places and situations that trigger these feelings.

This is how agoraphobia develops, but other phobias develop in a similar way. Some survivors do not feel safe when they are alone in case the feelings and memories about the abuse return.

SOCIAL PHOBIA

Social phobia is a fear of meeting people or being in situations where there are other people. Many survivors suffer from anxiety in social situations. They feel very self-conscious and think that other people are looking at them and judging them. This is not surprising, considering the shame many survivors feel about what has happened to them. Survivors often have negative thoughts that other people can see how guilty, dirty or bad they are inside, or can tell that they have been sexually abused.

Survivors often cope with the way the abuse has affected them by isolating themselves from other people, feeling uncomfortable around others. They may avoid other people because they are afraid of being harmed, abused or betrayed again. Some survivors have more specific fears in social situations; for example, they may feel particularly self-conscious when they are eating in public. Some people feel they have a lump in their throat or they are going to choke.

Joan was abused, on many occasions, by her sister's boyfriend in the bathroom and toilet of her parents' home, after which she had to go back into the sitting room and face her family. Each time, she felt ashamed and guilty, and felt sure her family would be able to tell what she had just been doing. As an adult, Joan was shy and self-conscious, often blushing and trying to avoid being the centre of attention. She was too embarrassed to go to the toilet when she was at work or in pubs and other public places, although she didn't understand why. When she came out of a public toilet, she thought everyone was staring at her. She felt guilty, anxious, embarrassed and unsteady on her feet. These were the same feelings and physical sensations that she had had when she came out of the toilet at home after she had been abused as a child. She avoided these emotions by drinking as little as possible when she was out so she would not need to go to the toilet. Eventually, she stopped going to the toilet all day at work and avoided going to pubs or other social gatherings. Joan started off with a specific fear of being seen leaving a toilet or bathroom, but this eventually developed into a more general social phobia, a generalized fear of many situations involving other people.

OBSESSIONAL PROBLEMS

People with high anxiety sometimes develop obsessional problems. They may feel they have to clean their house for hours every day; count things; do something a particular number of times; or check over and over again that the doors are locked. There are usually repetitive thoughts that go along with the actions – for example, 'If I don't check the door is locked six times, my son will have a terrible accident' or, 'If I don't clean the kitchen floor again, everyone will know how dirty I am.' Some people have repetitive thoughts but do not engage in repetitive action.

One way of coping with the anxiety and the memories of sexual abuse is to distract yourself by repeatedly doing something. While you are busy cleaning, counting or checking, you are distracted from thinking about the past and tend to feel less anxious for a little while. Survivors often cope with their bad feelings by cleaning; some wash their bodies over and over again in an attempt to feel clean. When survivors feel dirty or contaminated inside, they often try to make up for this by trying to keep their homes immaculately clean. They may spend many hours every day cleaning the house and be unable to leave a cup unwashed or a speck of dirt on the carpet.

> I have huge rows with my husband if he leaves anything on the floor. I always take my vacuum cleaner up to bed with me and sometimes I have to vacuum the whole house at four in the morning. **Pam**

Fiona was sexually and physically abused as a child. She felt dirty and was often nervous and afraid; she coped with these feelings by constantly cleaning her bedroom.

> When I was a child I used to scrub my bedroom at all times of the day. I felt dirty so I'd take up the carpet and scrub the floorboards and the walls. I was always cleaning. I'd even get up in the night and start sweeping my bedroom. **Fiona**

As an adult, Fiona continued to manage her emotions in this way.

> When I grew up and got my own house I was obsessed with cleaning. I'd start at 7 in the morning and still be at it at midnight. If I didn't half-kill myself cleaning, I felt bad and dirty so it was like a ritual, I cleaned to make myself feel better. **Fiona**

The more anxious a person with an obsessional problem feels, the more they clean, count or check to help them cope with the anxiety. Doing these things brings temporary relief, but this is soon followed by a feeling of even greater anxiety. When a survivor is anxious because he or she feels out of control or in danger, these repetitive thoughts and actions can be reassuring in the short term. They may also be a superstitious way of trying to ward off danger.

Fiona was in danger of sexual and physical violence throughout her childhood. As an adult, she still saw danger around her all the time and believed any happiness she had would be taken from her, just like in her childhood. When she was under stress, Fiona had obsessional thoughts about her daughter and husband being killed; she tried to ward off her fears by cleaning her house until it was spotless.

> I feel as if Amy and Andrew are going to be taken away from me. Every minute I'm with them seems to be the last. I can't enjoy them. I get flashes of them gone. The thoughts are different every day. One day it's Amy getting killed on her bike or being knocked down, the next it's they are both going to get killed in the car and another day it's the house is going to burn down. Everything around me feels dangerous. My obsession with cleaning the house is back and it has taken over this last week. **Fiona**

Obsessional problems start off as a way of coping but can become very debilitating and can be very hard to overcome by yourself. It may help if you follow the suggestions in this chapter to: reduce the level of your anxiety; write down and replace your irrational thoughts with more realistic ones as soon as they pop up; and try to avoid or reduce behaviours such as checking, cleaning and counting. If the thoughts and behaviours are extreme and take up a large part of your day, you may have OCD. If your symptoms are severe or badly affecting your life, your GP may be able to refer you for help. CBT can be very helpful for OCD.

Coping with anxiety and fears

If you are always worrying about what may happen in the future, it may help if you reduce your general level of anxiety by taking control of your physical symptoms, and write down your worrying thoughts and challenge them, as described below. If you experienced a great deal of fear in your childhood you may, as an adult, still feel tense and anxious. Trying not to think about your abuse can increase your anxiety; working through your feelings about your childhood abuse can help you to reduce your anxiety.

The fears a survivor experiences as an adult are often related to his or her fears as a child and to the situations in which he or she was abused. If you have a phobia or intense fear of certain situations, objects, people or animals, try to discover if there is a link between the fear or phobia and your abuse. Is there a connection between whatever frightens you now and your abuser, where the abuse occurred, what happened during the abuse or the threats the abuser used? Understanding the link between your specific fear and where it originates can help you reduce the fear. You may realize that you are afraid of bathrooms because you were abused in a bathroom, or you are phobic about knives because you were threatened with knives as a child. Some fears may have no obvious link with the abuse, yet the stress caused by the abuse probably played an important part in creating and maintaining the fear. After attending a survivors' group and working through her difficulties, Kate realized that her fear of men was linked to her abuse.

> I can handle men much better now. So much so that I recently took driving lessons with a male instructor and really enjoyed learning to drive. **Kate**

You have *learnt* to feel anxious and afraid because of your bad experiences. You can also learn how to reduce the bad feelings and live a normal life without excessive fear. People suffering with anxiety are often afraid they are going to lose control. You can overcome this fear by learning to gain self-control in situations that are usually frightening. The suggestions in the rest of this chapter can help you to reduce your symptoms of anxiety.

Learning to control your general anxiety should help reduce your fears and obsessions. If you are very anxious or have a phobia or obsession that is disrupting your life, ask your GP to refer you for expert help. It will help your GP refer you to the most appropriate specialist if you tell them about your past abuse or any other past traumas, but you do not need to tell your GP about the sexual abuse if that is too difficult for you. Look back at the list of anxiety symptoms in Box 6 and tick off any that you experience. In the following section, we suggest ways in which you can learn to deal with the three parts of anxiety: physical symptoms, negative thoughts and behaviours. If you have panic attacks, it is important that you first learn how to control them (see Appendix 1).

PHYSICAL SYMPTOMS

You can begin to control the physical symptoms of anxiety by learning how to relax, learning how to breathe correctly and taking exercise. When people are afraid, they tend to tense their muscles, and this can cause headaches, chest pains, stiffness or pain in almost any part of the body. If you are anxious, you are probably tensing up more and more as the day goes on. You need to find a way of relaxing your muscles. It may help to learn a relaxation exercise such as the kind taught in antenatal classes or at the end of a yoga class; these often consist of being verbally guided to relax each muscle group in turn (try looking for relaxation exercises on the internet). Mindfulness training and meditation can also be very useful in helping you let go and feel more in the moment – instead of worrying about what is going to happen in the future.

Remember, you have learnt to be tense, so you need to learn how to relax and let go of your tension again. Practise a relaxation exercise every day at first. When you feel generally less tense, you need only do the relaxation exercise three or four times a week and when you are feeling particularly stressed. When people have been tense for a long time, they sometimes feel strange when they begin to relax. Persevere and you will eventually become familiar and comfortable with the feeling of being relaxed.

For some people, gardening, running, knitting, yoga, meditation or cooking can be relaxing. Breathing exercises are also very good ways of relaxing. It is important that you choose a way of relaxing that suits you and try to relax completely every day. When you can relax, you will be able to learn to notice the first signs of tension and then let go and relax straight away before the tension builds up. Learning to relax will also help you sleep better.

Controlling your breathing

When we are afraid, the natural reaction is to breathe very fast or to gasp in air (hyperventilation) to get ourselves ready for action. We breathe in oxygen and breathe out carbon dioxide, and the bloodstream usually contains a balance between the two. Hyperventilation occurs when someone breathes too fast and breathes out too much carbon dioxide, creating an imbalance between oxygen and carbon dioxide in the blood. Many of the physical symptoms of anxiety are due to hyperventilation. Unfortunately, breathing too much makes you *feel* short of breath so you try to breathe even faster, creating a greater imbalance in your blood.

When you notice yourself becoming afraid, try to breathe very slowly and smoothly. Try closing your mouth and breathing through your nose, not your mouth at all – it's hard to breathe fast through your nose!

Overbreathing can become a habit so that people breathe too fast, or sigh a lot, even when they are not afraid. Practise breathing slowly and gently and become more aware of your breathing.

Appendix 1 describes how to breathe properly to take control of the physical symptoms of fear (it may be helpful for you to read Appendix 1 now, if you haven't already, so you can begin to take control of your breathing and anxiety).

Taking exercise

Your body increases the production of stress hormones when you are afraid. Residues of these stress hormones left in your body can leave you feeling restless and unable to sleep; exercise can help eliminate them from your bloodstream. Exercise has also been shown to change people's mood and help them feel better. 'Exercise' does not just mean going to the gym; it could be going for a brisk walk or doing some gardening. Regular exercise can help you to overcome some of the physical effects of your anxiety and fears.

CHALLENGING NEGATIVE THOUGHTS

Feeling afraid usually begins with negative thoughts about what is happening, what is about to happen or what other people are thinking. Sometimes the negative thoughts are triggered by noticing benign physical reactions, like palpitations, and thinking they are signs that something is wrong. A vicious circle begins with negative thoughts triggering physical symptoms of fear, which lead to more negative thoughts and so on. For some survivors, the fear may build up until they feel out of control and panicky or have a panic attack. You can break this vicious circle if you learn to talk yourself through your fear by replacing your usual negative thoughts with more realistic thoughts.

Here is an example of the thoughts of an anxious survivor who feels very nervous about going into a local shop. On the left are her usual negative thoughts (which increase her anxiety), and on the right are more realistic thoughts (which help her feel more in control of the situation).

Negative thoughts	*Realistic thoughts*
'Everyone is staring at me. They know there's something wrong with me. They think I'm dirty. My heart's going funny. They are looking at my children; they think my kids are scruffy and not looked after properly.'	'The people are not staring at me, they are just looking round. No one can see what I'm feeling. My heart is not going funny. It's only beating faster because I'm nervous. It won't do me any harm. No one knows I've been abused. They are only looking at my kids because they look so nice in their new coats. I'll just breathe slowly to calm myself down and I'll be all right. I'll buy the bread and go home for a cup of tea.'

Such negative thoughts are not realistic, and they make you feel more afraid. You may not realize you are having these negative thoughts and think that the fear just descends upon you. By becoming aware of your negative thoughts, and replacing these with more balanced appraisals, you can reduce your fear. Write down the thoughts that just seem to pop into your head when you notice that you are beginning to feel afraid, and then try to challenge these thoughts by writing down more realistic thoughts. In the same way, you can write down any worries that pop into your head and see if you can find more rational ways of thinking about the problem.

This will not be easy at first but it is a skill you can learn, and with practice you will reduce your negative thoughts and your anxiety. (Chapter 9, 'Depression and low self-esteem', contains more examples of how to challenge and replace negative thoughts.)

CHANGING WHAT YOU DO

No escaping

A very common response to fear is to want to leave the situation. As we said earlier, escaping from frightening situations may make you feel better immediately, but it can make you more anxious in the long run. The advice below only applies to situations where you are afraid but are not in any real danger. If you are in a situation where you may be harmed, you must leave for your own safety.

A key rule is DO NOT ESCAPE when you are feeling afraid (or are having a panic attack). Try to stay in the situation until your fear dies down. Find a quiet corner or sit down somewhere but try to stick it out. If you do feel that you have to leave, do this as slowly as you can, wait until you feel calmer and then return to the situation. Leave, if you want to, *after* your fear has died down. Remember, feeling anxious is very unpleasant but not harmful. By staying in the situation, you are learning that the fear will die down by itself.

Facing up to your fears

Once you have been frightened in a situation, you may avoid going into that situation again, and this will cause your fear to get worse. The next important rule is DO NOT AVOID. To defeat your fears, you need to face up to them. You can devise and work through a programme to help you overcome your fears. The first step is to find out exactly what situations trigger these fears. You need to be as specific as possible. It may be going out alone that frightens you.

It may be only supermarkets that frighten you, or only supermarkets when they are very busy. Try to define clearly exactly which situations increase your fear, including where it happens, when it happens and what people are around (or not around) when it happens.

Draw up a list of situations where you become frightened, and then put them in order from the least scary to the scariest. Start your list with a situation where you experience only a little fear (for example, going into the local shop when it is empty), and finish with your most feared situation (for example, going into a crowded supermarket alone on a busy Saturday afternoon). Try to include as many steps as possible between the least and the most frightening situations.

Begin by attempting the situation on your list that frightens you the least. Learn to take control of your fear by entering and staying in the situation, trying to relax, slowing your breathing and talking yourself through it by challenging your negative thoughts. You need to practise this every day. Notice if it gets easier.

When you can cope with the least difficult situation, move down your list and try the next task. Relax, breathe slowly, replace your negative thoughts and, step by step, face up to your feared situations.

You may find it easier to work through your programme on your own, or you may want to have someone with you when you first start practising, but aim to try the steps on your own when you can.

Feelings of fear or anxiety are sometimes triggered by things that can be avoided without interfering with your life too much. You may be able to avoid some triggers easily in the long term, whereas other triggers can be avoided in the short term as a means of stabilizing your emotions and gaining a sense of control until you have dealt with the underlying issues. You may find, for example, that watching programmes about child abuse, or listening to certain types of music, trigger flashbacks or anxiety attacks. Triggers such as these can usually be avoided fairly easily (turn the TV or radio off, or leave the room) until you feel more able to cope with them. You will find more about dealing with triggers in the *Breaking Free Workbook*.

Symptoms of trauma

As we discussed in Chapter 2, child sexual abuse is a traumatic experience or a series of traumatic experiences, and the symptoms of trauma are the result of overwhelming and unprocessed information becoming 'stuck' in the brain. These symptoms include flashbacks, nightmares, hallucinations, dissociation and hypervigilance (the body and brain being always on alert, being jumpy, looking round for danger); look at Box 2 in Chapter 2 for a list of symptoms of PTSD and trauma, and see how many apply to you. Flashbacks, nightmares, hallucinations and other symptoms are ways that the unprocessed information from the past 'leaks out' or expresses itself.

Contemporary research is exploring the links between childhood trauma and symptoms of psychosis (visual hallucinations, paranoia, hearing voices). People who have been sexually abused may have a ten times greater risk of experiencing hallucinations than people who have not been abused. This suggests that some of the symptoms of psychosis are created by trauma such as sexual abuse rather than by genetics or a biochemical disorder. The good news is that very effective treatments for the effects of trauma are now available. Having an episode of psychosis, or experiencing some of the other extreme symptoms resulting from abuse, can be traumatizing in itself.

NIGHTMARES

The traumatic events and emotions that have become 'stuck' in the circuits of the brain often come to the surface in the form of nightmares. Rachel felt so terrified by her nightmares that she made her fiancé walk the streets with her at night so she could avoid having to go to sleep. Nightmares often illustrate fears and memories that are too frightening or painful for survivors to face up to when they are conscious, but they are not necessarily an accurate picture of past events. Survivors often have nightmares about death, perhaps expressing the feeling that the sexual abuse had killed something in them, or resulting from their fears during the abuse that they would be killed. Remembering their own sexual abuse may make survivors anxious about the safety of their own children, and this may come out in bad dreams or nightmares.

My fears were really coming out in my nightmares. I dreamt that I was in town and suddenly realized that I had left my young daughter in someone's care where my abuser could get to her. I desperately tried to save her before he abused her. However fast I tried to go, I couldn't seem to reach her. The abuser was getting nearer to her all the time, right up to him opening the door to where she was, then I woke up screaming. **Kate**

Nightmares can be terrifying, but they can sometimes be a useful way for survivors to process their memories about the abuse, to express their fears and to explore more difficult feelings.

Coping with nightmares

Whenever I had a flashback or a nightmare, I would write it down and this really helped. **Polly**

Nightmares can be a way for your subconscious fears and memories to come into awareness. One way to deal with them is to write them down in detail afterwards so you become consciously aware of the underlying fears, instead of the fears being hidden in the back of your mind. Processing your memories about the abuse and working on your feelings about it will help you conquer your fears, and the nightmares will hopefully subside; see below for the best way to do this. Remember, though, that nightmares are not usually accurate memories of events.

HALLUCINATIONS – THE TRAUMA OF ABUSERS' THREATS
The threats used by abusers to silence children and young people can be so terrifying or life-threatening that the children develop lasting fears that the threats will be carried out. A child or young person can easily be traumatized when an abuser issues extreme threats in order to keep them quiet. The experience can be so over-whelming that it is impossible for anyone, especially a child, to understand and process the fear while it is happening. The threat therefore remains unprocessed, that is, 'stuck', in the brain along with all the feelings that were experienced at the time it was uttered. These unprocessed experiences and emotions contribute to a feeling that the threat is still active now and is about to be carried out.

Sophie was raped on a gravestone when she was only 7 years old. The abuser said that if she told anyone, the rotting man in the grave below her would know and would find her. This threat was so terrifying that Sophie was overwhelmed with horror and blocked off all memory of the abuse for a while (that is, she dissociated from the sexual assault and threatening situation). As an adult, Sophie had nightmares about rotting bodies coming to get her and a phobia of dead bodies. The unprocessed terror from the trauma left Sophie feeling as if the threat was still active and she was in danger of it coming true at any time.

Lorna's abuser said he would know, and would kill her, if she ever told anyone about the abuse. This threat was so frightening to Lorna that she was traumatized by the threat itself and remained extremely anxious for many years afterwards. She felt unable to talk to anyone about the sexual abuse because, if she ever tried to talk about it, she would see the abuser in the room with her, could hear him threatening to kill her and believed the threat would be carried out.

Holly was raped many times on an extended visit to family members in the USA when she was 13 years old. The abuser kept a gun under the pillow as a threat to make her cooperate with the abuse, and to keep her quiet about what was happening. The abuser told Holly that he would not only kill her if she disclosed the abuse, but would also kill the person she told. When Holly first disclosed to me, she became frozen with terror when she saw her abuser in the clinic room, standing next to me and threatening me with a gun. This example demonstrates that trauma-based hallucinations are different from flashbacks. The abuser never held a gun to my head in real life, so her experience was not a flashback (the experience of reliving aspects of an actual event). Holly's hallucination was an activation of traumatic material left unprocessed since the threats were originally uttered, resulting in the client believing and perceiving that the threat was about to be carried out.

Many survivors hallucinate their abusers. They can see, hear and smell the abuser, or sense the abuser is in the room with them, when the abuser is not actually there, or even after the abuser has died. Half of the Wakefield survivors have had the experience of seeing their abusers when they were not actually there. In our experience with survivors, these trauma-based hallucinations are not related to the severity of the *acts* involved in the abuse, but occur when the abuser had traumatized the children with horrific *threats.* When the unprocessed terror, laid down when the threat was initially issued, is triggered, the survivor believes that the abuser is actually back in the room with him or her, and about to carry out the threat.

Coping with hallucinations

To *eliminate* hallucinations, the underlying terror needs to be processed using trauma-focused therapies (see 'Summary and suggestions' below). The *Breaking Free Workbook* contains more information and ways of *managing* hallucinations to help you cope in the present. The following technique is from the *Workbook* and is very effective in giving you control over trauma-based hallucinations of the abuser.

When a survivor hallucinates the abuser (or hallucinates objects, like knives, connected with the threat that was used), the abuser is not actually there, even though the survivor strongly believes the abuser is in the room and has a very strong perception or sense that the abuser is real and present. If this happens to you, try the following technique: when the hallucination of the abuser appears, throw a harmless object like a screwed-up paper towel or a foam ball at the place where you see the abuser. Amazingly, the image/abuser will suddenly disappear. This is quite a surprise when you first see it happen and, in our experience, it always works with trauma-based hallucinations. In fact, you can throw anything light and harmless – a foam ball works just as well as a hard object, which could cause damage to property or other people. Please do not put yourself or other people in danger by throwing hard objects.

The hallucination of the abuser will also disappear immediately if you wave an arm through the spot where the abuser appears to be. Your brain knows that you cannot throw a paper towel or wave your arm through a person who is really there; it cannot sustain the image of the abuser as real when an object passes through it, so the image just disappears. Knowing you can get rid of an hallucination of the abuser by yourself can help you feel more powerful and no longer controlled by the abuser. If you are initially too scared to try this yourself, ask a friend or therapist to do it for you. Seeing that this technique really works may give you confidence to try it for yourself.

Coping with trauma symptoms

Sexual abuse is a traumatic experience, and some of your symptoms may be a result of frightening material that is still 'stuck' in your brain's information-processing system. It is not easy to eliminate these symptoms using anxiety management techniques – trauma-focused therapies are more effective. If you suffer with flashbacks, hallucinations, nightmares, hypervigilance, dissociation or other symptoms of trauma; you will benefit from some trauma-focused therapy. EMDR therapy and trauma-focused CBT (see 'Getting help with trauma or PTSD symptoms' in Chapter 15, 'Overcoming the problems') will help you process the overwhelming feelings and experiences, and reduce your trauma symptoms. EMDR is also very effective in eliminating phobias and the physical symptoms resulting from trauma, such as hypervigilance/hyperarousal.

A note on medication

You may be taking tranquillizers or antidepressants to help you with your anxiety. These drugs can sometimes help in the short term by suppressing your symptoms, but in the long term you will probably need to face up to your fears to defeat them. The techniques described here may help you in time to control your anxiety symptoms without taking any tablets. DO NOT STOP TAKING ANY TABLETS SUDDENLY – this can be very dangerous. If you want to reduce your medication, please discuss this with your doctor.

Summary and suggestions

- The experience of childhood sexual abuse, and the associated feelings of fear and dread, often result in the adult survivor having symptoms of anxiety, and sometimes leaves them suffering with specific fears, phobias or obsessions. Your level of anxiety will decrease after you work through your feelings about the abuse. You would probably benefit from working on some of the symptoms of anxiety now to help you cope while you work through your past experiences.
- To overcome anxiety, it is necessary to face up to your fears and work on your physical symptoms, negative thoughts and behaviours. You have learnt to be anxious and fearful because of your

childhood experiences. You *can* learn to overcome your fears and take control of your own life again. Try following the steps outlined in the 'Coping with anxiety and fears' section above. Practise some form of relaxation (or mindfulness or meditation) and breathing exercise every day.

- If your symptoms of fear or anxiety are disrupting your life, see your GP and discuss this with him or her. Ask for a referral to someone who can help with anxiety management or relaxation (or who works with childhood sexual abuse if you are ready). See 'Sources of help' at the back of this book.

- Flashbacks, hallucinations, nightmares, hypervigilance, dissociation and other symptoms of trauma are best eliminated with trauma-focused therapies such as EMDR and trauma-focused CBT; see Chapter 15, 'Overcoming the problems'. Remember to use the technique described earlier in the chapter to help you manage any visual hallucinations you may experience.

- Appendix 1 describes how to breathe properly to help you control your anxiety symptoms and how to manage panic attacks.

- The first chapter in the *Breaking Free Workbook* has more ideas on 'How to keep safe.' The chapters on 'Coping strategies' and 'Dealing with emotions, flashbacks and hallucinations' in the *Workbook* may also be helpful. The latter chapter includes techniques for managing hallucinations of the abuser and also looks at identifying, monitoring and dealing with triggers.

9

Depression and low self-esteem

How I wish I had sought help long before I did. I can remember feeling isolated, guilty and having little self-esteem from as far back as I can remember. I had no idea that my grim view of life and low opinion of myself were linked to my sexual abuse.
Joanne

Survivors often have a low opinion of themselves and lack self-confidence and self-esteem. They may feel worthless, useless and unlovable. Many survivors put on a 'front' and present themselves as capable, cheerful and confident, while feeling wretched inside. Survivors may be so overwhelmed by their low opinion of themselves and lack of confidence that they suffer bouts of depression. Depression immobilizes people, making them unable to act positively or find pleasure in things. This in turn further undermines self-confidence and starts a vicious circle of decreasing self-esteem and increasing depression. This chapter looks at low self-esteem and depression, the connections between them and childhood sexual abuse and what can be done to overcome them.

Low self-esteem

If children have a loving and supportive environment, they develop self-confidence and self-esteem as they grow up. They learn:

- to trust their own judgement;
- to feel 'safe' in the world;
- that they can be liked for themselves;
- that they can make their own decisions;
- that they are valuable;
- that they deserve to be treated with love and respect.

Children and young people learn these things if they are around others who love and protect them, and yet allow them the freedom to develop in their own way and to make mistakes. When these children become adults, they are less likely to become depressed because their secure childhoods have given them confidence and made them feel positive about themselves.

What happens, though, to children who have been sexually abused? They might learn:

- not to trust their own judgement (the person they trusted betrayed them);
- to believe the world is a dangerous place where trusted people take advantage of them and use them for their own ends;
- that they are only liked when they do what the abuser wants them to do, and that they are not accepted for themselves;
- that they are controlled by other people and cannot decide for themselves who can touch their body;
- that they are not valued for themselves, and that what they feel doesn't matter;
- that they deserve to be abused and to have their wishes disregarded.

Such experiences have the effect of undermining children's self-confidence and self-esteem, making them more likely to feel bad about themselves and go on to suffer from depression when they become adults.

Lucy and Jocelyn describe how they felt about themselves as children.

> After the nightmare of being raped and sexually attacked by my uncle and dad, I lost my self-esteem. I felt shy and had no self-confidence. I was frightened and I hated myself. I felt I could never please my mum and dad and always felt second best. **Lucy**

> My self-confidence was very low, I thought everyone was better than me. I couldn't think of anything I was good at. I could think of scores of things I was bad at. I was nervous, frightened, always tense and I always had tummy ache. I never said what I wanted, what I would like. I didn't think anyone was interested or really wanted to know. I didn't know who I was, what I wanted, and I felt I had no voice. I was letting events and other people carry me along. I was not in control. I was on a conveyor belt and I couldn't get off. **Jocelyn**

Like Lucy and Jocelyn, many survivors grow up feeling inferior and lacking in self-confidence. They may feel so worthless and unacceptable that they put on a 'front' to other people and never allow their real feelings and thoughts to be known.

> When I left school, I had no confidence in myself and I found it very hard making relationships because of what had happened to me. I thought I was some kind of pervert. I am still very shy when I meet people for the first time and I seem to put a barrier around myself. **Anthony**

Survivors may strive for the approval and love they feel unworthy of, by always looking after and trying to please other people. Many survivors seek approval in order to feel acceptable and think any form of rejection is devastating proof that they are unacceptable and unlovable. Lack of self-confidence and self-esteem can lead to problems such as:

- not being able to say 'no' to people;
- not being able to ask for things;
- always putting other people's needs first;
- believing it doesn't matter what you feel or what you want;
- not being spontaneous;
- not being able to make decisions;
- waiting to see what happens, rather than making a choice;
- acting passively;
- staying in bad relationships;
- letting people take advantage;
- feeling guilty;
- feeling obliged to do things;
- a feeling of having no choice or control;
- hiding real feelings;
- not being able to express opinions;
- feeling let down by people;
- feeling helpless;
- compulsively caring for other people, putting yourself last.

When children and young people are being sexually abused, they usually cannot fight back or stop the abuse. They are powerless in relation to the abuser and learn to passively accept the abuse, remain silent and keep their feelings to themselves. The child learns that the abuser's feelings and needs are more important than his or her own. The survivors' opinions and feelings don't count; they have no rights; and they learn over time to passively accept whatever people do to them. Many survivors grow up continuing to keep their feelings of anger and distress inside and passively accepting abuse from other people.

> I was so used to being used. I didn't know I had a right to free will and choice about how I wanted to live my life, so I married an abusive man when I was 17. In many ways, he was like my brother (the abuser), he abused me verbally, battered me and intimidated me by smashing up the furniture. His threats to kill me became almost routine. I accepted my fate without rebellion for many years. I did not like my husband, yet if I had to describe my feelings during all those abusive years the only word that comes to my mind is 'numb'. I was indeed passive. **Ingrid**

Survivors who always put other people's feelings and needs before their own, and never stand up for themselves, are likely to be used and abused again as adults. They may also be prone to occasional aggressive outbursts when the bottled-up feelings can no longer be held back. They then hate themselves for losing control and feel even more guilty and frightened. Passive behaviour can make people feel more helpless and worthless, and makes them more likely to become depressed.

Depression

Depression can be a very disturbing and frightening experience. People often feel that depression descends upon them from nowhere, and they feel powerless to understand or change how they are feeling. It can cause physical changes such as tiredness and loss of appetite, but depression is not primarily a physical problem. Depression is rooted in people's past experiences; their thoughts and feelings about themselves and the world; and the ways they have learnt to cope. Depression can be broken down into three parts: depressed feelings, depressed thoughts, and depressed behaviour (see Box 7).

Box 7 Depressed thoughts, feelings and behaviour

Depressed thoughts include thoughts about being:
- punished
- useless
- unable to control situations or alter them

- disliked
- unwanted
- worthless and unlovable
- stupid
- a failure
- a destructive person
- always used and abused
- ugly and repulsive
- fat.

Also, bad thoughts about:
- death
- illness
- accidents
- catastrophes
- life being pointless.

Depressed feelings include emotions such as:
- sadness
- feeling like a failure
- guilt
- shame
- self-hatred
- anger
- dissatisfaction
- hopelessness
- worry
- feeling out of control
- feeling overwhelmed
- helplessness
- feeling numb.

Depressed behaviour includes:
- crying a lot or being unable to cry
- withdrawing and avoiding people
- eating less than usual
- staying in bed
- drinking alcohol, overeating or taking drugs
- watching TV all day
- doing very little
- not getting dressed, not washing regularly and not looking after self
- not being able to sleep or waking up early
- being unable to make decisions or do simple tasks.

DEPRESSED THOUGHTS AND FEELINGS

Children and young people who have been sexually abused often believe that they are worthless, inferior, useless, disgusting, unacceptable or unlovable. They believe these things because of the way they have been treated, and sometimes because the abuser, or someone else, has told them this directly. By the time these children become adults, they have already had years of practice in thinking negatively about themselves and often about the world in general.

> I didn't care about myself. I hated everything about myself and there wasn't one good thing I could say about myself. I blamed myself for everything. **Rhys**

These negative or depressed thoughts become habits, automatic ways of thinking that survivors may not even be conscious of, and that lead on to depressed emotions.

Some survivors have had bouts of depression since childhood. Others may become depressed as adults because an everyday upset, such as being rejected in a relationship or not getting promoted at work, reactivates their underlying negative thoughts and feelings about themselves.

DEPRESSED BEHAVIOUR

Depressed thoughts and feelings cause physical changes in people's bodies and affect their behaviour. Some people feel constantly tired or lethargic when they are depressed. Others feel agitated and unable to sleep or eat. Some people are unable to cry when they are depressed, whereas others become very tearful. People also change their behaviour when they are depressed in order to cope with their bad feelings. Drinking, overeating, sleeping, taking drugs and self-injury are all ways of trying to blot out negative feelings and thoughts.

> I turned to alcohol to try and block out the past but it just made the flashbacks worse. Then I started suffering from depression. That's when I started to harm myself, because I didn't feel clean and I felt I had betrayed my body. I would be hostile and abusive to the staff in the casualty department. I didn't mean them any harm, because I can't say I'm violent, but I am short-tempered and sometimes I do feel isolated from people who just can't seem to understand me. **Anthony**

Depressed people tend to withdraw and avoid other people because they feel so worthless and unacceptable. They may attempt suicide to escape from their painful feelings or because they feel so helpless and hopeless about the future.

All these behaviours tend to make the negative thoughts and feelings worse. A drinking or eating binge temporarily blocks out bad feelings, but then leads to feelings of guilt, self-hatred and hopelessness.

Depressed behaviour makes people more likely to have negative thoughts and feelings, and this in turn makes them more likely to behave in a depressed way. Unless this vicious circle is broken, the depression becomes worse and worse.

Overcoming depression and low self-esteem

Reading through this book and working on your thoughts and feelings about your abuse will help you build up your self-esteem and feel less depressed. You will begin to feel more self-confident and worthwhile as you start to feel less guilty and ashamed, and stop blaming yourself for being abused. As you begin to feel better about yourself, your depression will be easier to overcome. Talking to other people, especially other survivors, or seeing a therapist can also be helpful.

> I have felt lonely and isolated. Being able to discuss how I feel with people and being more open about myself is a great help.
> **Anthony**

When you feel depressed, it is often extremely difficult to believe that you will ever feel any differently. Nothing seems to help, and other people's suggestions can seem impossible to carry out. Feeling so hopeless and beyond help is part of being depressed. Fiona has now overcome her depression but can remember how hopeless she previously felt.

> I can't put into words how much I hurt. The darkness, the emptiness and the feeling of hopelessness were unbearable. I never thought I'd get through it and even when it did start to lift, I was frightened of going back there. As I write this and remember the pain I can't stop the tears, but there is no fear because I know now I'll never be like that again. **Fiona**

Try to remember that people can and do overcome depression. Below we suggest ways of tackling your depressed behaviour and thoughts and becoming more assertive. Take things one step at a time. Don't expect too much too soon. Try to be pleased and reward yourself for any positive changes you make, however small. Don't be harsh with yourself if you don't change as quickly as you would like to.

CHANGING DEPRESSED BEHAVIOUR

Depressed behaviour is not only a reaction to depression, it also causes the depression to worsen. You can start to break the vicious circle of depression by making some changes in your behaviour. It may be hard to get started if you are feeling hopeless. Take it one step at a time. Set yourself easy tasks you can achieve and feel good about. See if you can work on some of the points given below.

- Get up at a reasonable time rather than staying in bed and then feeling guilty. Reward yourself for getting up and start the day with some positive thoughts (see the section below on affirmations).
- Take some exercise. Exercise helps people feel better both physically and mentally. Try walking, gardening, dancing, yoga or swimming, whatever exercise suits you. Try to do some exercise *every day* – just going for a walk around the local area will help.
- Try to eat regular meals even if you have little appetite. Choose good, healthy food to give you energy to tackle your problems. If you are overeating, read Chapter 10 on eating problems and do the exercises that are suggested there. Overeating is often a way of covering up bad feelings and seeking comfort.
- Plan at least one thing every day that you enjoy – for example, have a bath, listen to music, play with your dog or cat, meditate, meet a friend for coffee or go to see a movie. If you can't think of anything that you find enjoyable at the moment, try doing something that you used to enjoy.
- Try to make some contact with people again, even if it is only for a short time. Avoiding people only increases thoughts that you are lonely and unlovable. Being with friends can help you begin to think and feel more positively – there are things to enjoy in life; people do like you; you are not alone.

Changing your behaviour is only the first step towards overcoming depression. It is also important to work on changing your negative or automatic thoughts.

CHALLENGING NEGATIVE THOUGHTS

Depression may *seem* to come out of the blue, but it is brought on and maintained by negative thoughts, often triggered by things you hear or see. Negative thinking affects your mood. Trying to recognize your negative thoughts and then challenging them, by questioning whether these thoughts are realistic, helps you to reduce your feelings of depression. Negative thoughts happen automatically and can be difficult to identify so you will need to persevere with the exercise below. Before attempting this exercise read through the instructions and the examples.

Exercise

Draw a line down the middle of a piece of paper and head one side 'negative thoughts' and the other side 'realistic thoughts'. Notice what negative thoughts are running through your head, particularly if you suddenly begin to feel worse. Write the thoughts down under the heading 'negative thoughts'. Write them down exactly as they go through your head in the first person and present tense (for example, 'I'm stupid'). Remember that it is the thoughts, not the feelings, that you are trying to recognize. For example, don't write, 'I was sitting feeling depressed and thinking about the future.' Write the exact thoughts – for example, 'I'll never feel any better. I'm going to be miserable for the rest of my life. There's no point in living.'

Next ask yourself, are these thoughts really true? Is there another way of seeing the situation, or of explaining what has happened, or of seeing yourself? Write down these alternative, more realistic, thoughts on the other side of the paper. The negative thoughts may seem realistic to you at the moment because you are depressed. Try to be *objective* and look at the evidence for and against your negative thoughts. If you cannot think of any more realistic thoughts, ask someone to help you. Keep a paper and pen at hand and write down your negative thoughts whenever they occur, or type them into a notes page on your smartphone, tablet or computer. Be sure to write the thoughts down rather than trying to do this exercise in your head. This exercise also needs to be done regularly over a period of time. Negative thinking builds up over years and it takes time to break the habit completely, but you may begin to feel a bit better quite quickly.

Aim to write down your negative thoughts in simple statements.

Example

Negative thoughts	Realistic thoughts
'I deserve to be abused.'	'No one deserves to be abused. I deserve to be treated with love and respect, like any other human being.'
'I am a complete failure.'	'I am not a complete failure. I have survived being abused and brought up my children, who are well looked after.'
'I am useless.'	'I am not useless. I sometimes make mistakes, just like everyone else.'
'I will never feel any better.'	'Feeling better takes time and effort. I have made the first step by reading this book and facing my problems. The survivors in this book have overcome their problems and so can I.'

Every time Fiona felt depressed, she stayed in bed. This gave her more opportunity to slip into thinking negatively about herself and her future. These thoughts happened automatically. She wasn't even aware of all the negative thoughts that were running through her head and making her feel even worse. Fiona decided to challenge her negative thoughts to help lift her depression. For the first time, she began to see that there were alternative ways of seeing herself and her situation.

Negative thoughts	Realistic thoughts
'I caused my parents and others to treat me the way they did by being disruptive. It was all my fault.'	'No, it wasn't my fault. I learnt to behave like that. I wasn't born disruptive. Circumstances and situations made me like that. I was crying out for help. I had

	bottled up my anger, frustration, fear and disgust about my neglect and abuse. I need not fear anything. I will handle whatever life dishes out. I am going to enjoy life now and get stronger so I can use my experience to help others, which I know I can do.'
'I'm dirty and my house always looks dirty.'	'I am not dirty. I am as good as anyone else. My house is not perfectly clean the way I wish it could be, like the ones on the TV. No one can be that clean if there are people and pets living in it comfortably. My house is clean and tidy, a lot cleaner than some and not as spotless as others, but then it is not a showhome. It is a home where people live and are comfortable.'
'I'm not as good as other people.'	'I'm just as good as the next person, if not better. I'm a very caring person and love my family. I haven't done a bad job in raising Amy, keeping a home and getting educated, even though I've had a hard life and suffered sexual abuse. I am going to try to like myself.'

Over the weeks, Fiona began to see that her negative thoughts were not realistic. She had got into the habit of thinking badly about herself because of how she had been treated as a child. Fiona began to see that there were many good things about herself. She had survived abuse and had made a new life for herself and was trying to overcome her problems. As a result, she began to accept herself and feel more powerful.

AFFIRMATIONS
Affirmations are positive statements about yourself. They help to remind you that you have good points and so increase your

feelings of self-confidence and self-esteem. They also help by coun-teracting negative thoughts. Affirmations can help in the journey towards overcoming depression and in stopping depression from developing.

Exercise

Write down three positive things about yourself. They could be things you like about yourself or are good at or are getting better at. If you can't think of anything yourself, ask a friend to help you.

Examples

I am good at my job.
I am courageous in facing my problems by reading this book.
I am getting to like and accept myself more every day.
I am a good listener.
I am a creative person and good at making things.
I am a keen gardener.
I like the way I keep on trying.

Say your positive statements every day before you get up. Write them on a piece of paper and stick them on cupboards, mirrors and so on where you will see them regularly. Put them on the notes page of your smartphone and remind yourself of them regularly.

CONFIDENCE-BUILDING OR ASSERTION TRAINING

Assertion training is a powerful way to increase self-esteem and can help in overcoming depression. It teaches that everyone has rights and that they can learn to think, feel and act positively by respecting their own rights and those of other people. Assertion training distinguishes four different types of behaviour.

- **Assertive** expressing feelings openly and honestly. Not allowing yourself to be used and put down, and not using or putting down anyone else.
- **Passive** not saying how you feel. Putting other people's feelings and rights before your own. Putting yourself down ('I am stupid') and allowing other people to use you.
- **Aggressive** putting your own feelings before anyone else's feel-ings. Using and putting down other people ('You are stupid'). Shouting and being physically aggressive.

- **Indirect** trying to get your own way without appearing to do so. Putting down other people while appearing to be friendly on the surface. Lying, being sarcastic, 'guilt-tripping' others, making excuses and being manipulative.

Most people behave in all these different ways at some point, but they usually have one style of behaviour that is more common than the others. Many survivors behave passively most of the time, and indirectly some of the time, and have occasional aggressive outbursts. Very few survivors have had opportunity to learn how to be assertive. It may help you feel stronger if you can find an assertion or confidence-building course, or a good book with exercises you can follow to help you become more assertive (see the book list 'Further reading' on the DABS website, given in the 'Sources of help' section at the back of this book).

Assertion training is usually more useful for survivors in the later stages of recovery. In the following account, Katarina shows how assertion has helped her.

Since I went to an assertion class, I have stopped accepting the blame and apologizing for everything that goes wrong in the lives of my family and other people. Before, I truly believed that everything was somehow my fault. Even if I was not directly involved, somehow I found a connection, a link that printed GUILT, BLAME, SHAME in capital letters in my mind. Now I realize I am not responsible for my family's happiness. I can love them and care for them, but ultimately they must create their own happiness. I cannot keep all unhappy experiences or problems from them.

As I refused to feel guilty any more, I understood that assertion is about how you value yourself. It is not right for me to treat other people better than I treat myself. I became more understanding, more forgiving and accepting of myself. I can see my faults and shortcomings but as I can accept them in others, I don't need to be perfect either.

Assertion has done something else for me. It has finally released me from this terrible need to put up the front of being 'superwoman', the one who can cope with everything and anything without getting tired or stressed. Too many people and things were eating away at my time and energy. There was not enough left for myself. So, I decided to change my life. I ignored the rooms with no wallpaper on their walls and I sat down in a chair and did nothing for an hour. It was the first time that I'd sat still without feeling guilty because there were other things to do. Then I made a list of my priorities and decided only to do the things that were really necessary or important to me.

The conscious decision to say 'I don't have time for this' or 'I feel tired' lifted enormous stress off me. I relaxed and found peace again. I have now gone back to doing some things that I gave up for a short while. But now I do it because I want to and not because I have to. This is the big difference in my life. **Katarina**

Fiona's coping methods

After suffering with depression most of my childhood and adult life, at 29 years of age I am now living. I know I have a long way to go but I no longer suffer from depression like I did. I still get a little down, but who doesn't? I see life differently now. I'm interested in lots of things whereas before I used to think 'What's the point?' Now I am trying to make up for those lost years, enjoying life and getting as much out of it as I can. I am now able to love my family dearly and to accept love. **Fiona**

Fiona tackled her depression by changing her behaviour (she made herself get up earlier, eat regularly and start seeing people socially again) and by challenging her negative thoughts. She realized she had got into the habit of lying in bed for hours and thinking badly about herself, and this was making her feel depressed. Fiona also went to an assertion group and began to express her feelings and change her behaviour. As she began to respect her own rights and feelings, and those of other people, her self-respect and self-confidence grew.

At the same time, Fiona was working in therapy on her memories and feelings about being sexually abused as a child. As she began to see she was not to blame for the abuse, she stopped feeling guilty and ashamed, understood more about her past behaviour, and began to feel more acceptable and worthwhile. Fiona had felt helpless and hopeless about ever feeling any better, but she overcame her depression. She started to feel better about herself and more hopeful about the future, and had renewed interest in life. Fiona regained her own strength and power, and you can too.

Suggestions

- Begin to change your depressed thoughts, feelings and behaviours, by following the suggestions and exercises in the chapter.
- There are many books on assertion and building up self-esteem in the 'Recovery' section of the DABS book list (at: <www.dabs.uk.com>).
- Attend a class on assertion or confidence-building or form your own group with friends.
- There are many useful videos on YouTube – type 'Assertiveness' or 'Confidence' into the search box. Be selective!
- The *Breaking Free Workbook* has chapters on 'Coping strategies' and 'Dealing with emotions, flashbacks and hallucinations' that may be helpful to you.
- If you are seriously depressed or the depression is affecting your life, please seek some help for yourself – you deserve it (see the 'Sources of help' section at the back of this book).

10

Eating problems and body image

When I became a teenager, I wanted to look pretty. I lost some weight, I looked like all the other girls. Yet when I looked in the mirror I only saw a fat girl, so ugly that I felt like apologizing every time someone had to look at me. I only saw myself with my brother's eyes. **Katarina**

The difficulty was, how to get thin? I couldn't diet because I ate for comfort. I ate to stop myself thinking, to keep the fears at bay. So I carried on eating and simply vomited the food straight back up. I ate when I felt bad about myself, then vomited. I gave in to sexual demands because I needed affection and reassurance. Then I'd feel bad about being promiscuous, so I'd eat. As the bulimia spiralled out of control I learnt to feel guilty about that too. When I was sexually assaulted as an adult, I ate as a way of coping. I ate because I felt angry about the abuse. I hated myself because I couldn't stop it happening. I ate because I had no control over my body. I ate because I felt angry that other people felt they had a right to hit me, to abuse me. But most of all I ate because I was afraid I deserved the abuse. I vomited because I could not hold so much pain, so much fear, so much hate and so much anger within myself and I could find no other way of letting it out. **Shirley**

In Western society, the pressures on women to remain slim, together with their responsibilities to provide food, result in women being more likely to have problems with body image and eating than men. Many women have a poor body image and are concerned about their weight, and some develop eating disorders. An eating problem is called an *eating disorder* when a person's behaviours and beliefs around food and the regulation of body weight are severe enough that he or she would receive a medical diagnosis if they were assessed by a psychiatrist or other medical practitioner.

In the past, it was believed that eating disorders were experienced almost exclusively by women, but a growing number of young men now have difficulties with their weight and with their body image. At least 10 per cent of people with eating disorders are male, but this is probably an underestimate as men are less likely to disclose difficulties with eating and body size, and professionals are less likely to look for the signs in men and boys. The rate of reporting eating problems in boys and men has recently doubled, and the latest figures estimate that perhaps 25 per cent of young people with eating disorders are male.

Survivors of sexual abuse are even more likely to have problems with their body image and eating. Survivors are often left with a dislike or even a hatred of their own bodies, which usually focuses on their weight, size or shape. They may dislike all of their bodies or just certain parts like their stomach, genitals, chest or hips. Many survivors do not like getting undressed in public changing rooms, do not like their partners to see them with no clothes on, and often avoid looking at their own bodies. It is not surprising that survivors feel particularly bad about their bodies because during sexual abuse the body is invaded and treated without respect.

This dislike of the body often leads to attempts to change it by repeated dieting, usually interspersed with periods of breaking the diet and overeating. Survivors frequently turn to eating when they are upset or angry and find it difficult to eat in a 'normal' way. Dieting and overeating can develop into a way for individuals to cope with bad feelings about themselves and what has happened to them.

What is an eating problem?

Many women, and a growing number of men, have problems with food and eating. People with eating problems are overconcerned or preoccupied with their body size, weight and shape. Women are often self-conscious about feeling overweight. They may weigh themselves every day and feel their mood change according to the reading on the scales. They may not want to go out of the house if their weight has increased or they feel fat. Men are more likely to worry about being too small and thin, having a puny chest or a lack of muscles. Both men and women with eating problems feel that life would be a lot better if they were a different size or shape. These feelings often lead to constant attempts to diet, to body-build or to use other ways of trying to control and transform their bodies. Men, or women, who are trying to build up muscle mass may also take chemical supplements to boost their size.

Unfortunately, when people try to keep to a strict diet, they often end up breaking the diet and overeating when they are under stress. Instead of eating when they are hungry, eating becomes a response to stress, bad feelings or difficult events in their lives. Eating can *temporarily* ease uncomfortable feelings.

If people eat according to their own strict rules about what and when they can eat, instead of in response to their body signals, they end up no longer knowing whether they are hungry or not. At times, everyone eats in response to how they are feeling (agitated, lonely, upset) rather than because they are hungry, but for most people eating does not become their main way of dealing with bad feelings. For some people, however, their focus on controlling their eating and body size can develop into an eating disorder, which can take over their lives and prevent them from dealing with the underlying causes of their problems. The main problems people have around food and eating are described below.

Binge-eating

Many people feel out of control around food and eat in response to bad feelings or to avoid feeling anything at all. Some people eat huge amounts of food very quickly and don't stop eating until they can physically eat no more – this is called binge-eating. During a binge, the food is not usually chewed or tasted but is quickly swallowed down. This is accompanied by a feeling of being out of control. The foods most commonly eaten in a binge are those that people usually try to avoid eating when they are on a diet, such as chocolate, biscuits, bread and other high-calorie foods. Binge-eating may temporarily lift people's mood, but afterwards they feel depressed, guilty about overeating and disgusted with themselves.

People who binge-eat often do not like to eat, or to eat much, in public and usually eat alone. Perhaps 10 per cent of young women in their late teens or early twenties binge-eat, although for many it will be a passing phase; a growing number of young men also binge-eat. Anyone who binge-eats at least once a week for 3 months may be diagnosed as having binge-eating disorder (BED) – this is the most common of the eating disorders.

Purging and other compensatory behaviours

Many people try to stick to a strict diet to control their weight but then, almost inevitably, break their diets and some will go on to binge-eat. After the binge, they feel disgusted with themselves and panic that they will gain weight and become fat, and feel they have to find a way of getting rid of all the calories as soon as possible. Some people return to restricting their food intake, but others use more drastic ways of trying to prevent any weight gain after a binge. They may immediately make themselves vomit up all the food; take large amounts of laxatives, diet pills or diuretics; or exercise excessively. These are all attempts to eliminate the extra calories and keep their weight down, and are called compensatory behaviours. For many, this purging is also a self-punishment for losing control and overeating.

This dieting–bingeing–purging cycle is called bulimia nervosa and can be very debilitating and medically dangerous. People with behaviours that could lead to a diagnosis of bulimia nervosa are usually very ashamed of the binge-eating and purging and keep it hidden from others. Their body weight is usually within the normal range. Research studies have found that being sexually abused as a child is a risk factor for developing bulimia in young women: they are much more likely to develop bulimia than young women who have not been abused.

Some people purge or use the other compensatory behaviours but do not binge-eat. This is also medically dangerous. Anyone who is binge-eating and/or purging should try to get some professional support to help them take control of their eating and purging cycle before it starts to have some physical and medical consequences.

Restricting food intake

Many people try to restrict their food intake to help them reduce their weight and to cope with the way they feel. Some people go to extreme lengths and try to eat very little or nothing at all. Anorexia nervosa is diagnosed when individuals have a significantly low body weight, a fear of being fat or gaining weight, and a distorted view of their body size and of their condition; for example, they may think eating one meal will make them fat, or they may deny that having a significantly low weight is unhealthy.

Some people with anorexia nervosa control their weight by severe restriction of what they eat; others will also binge-eat and then purge themselves or use other compensatory behaviours.

Many young women go through a phase of restricting their food intake and losing weight, but true anorexia nervosa is relatively uncommon; it makes up approximately 10 per cent of eating disorders. Boys and men also diet and restrict their food intake at times and can be diagnosed with anorexia nervosa, but this is less common than in women. Anorexia nervosa has serious, and sometimes fatal, health consequences so please get some help if you are severely restricting your food intake or are purging.

Even if you do not have a serious eating disorder, you may feel uncomfortable with your own body and the way you eat. If you are unhappy about your eating habits, the ideas and exercises in this chapter may help you understand more about why you eat or why you try to restrict your eating. Over time, they may help you develop a more 'normal' relationship with your body and your food intake. If your eating problem is disrupting your life or you feel unable to take control of your eating (or restricted eating), seek some professional help.

Eating problems – the background context

> As a teenager, I learnt that being thin, looking acceptable on the outside, gained me a sort of approval and praise, it gave me some self-esteem, although not enough to rid me of the fear that I was a 'bad' or 'unworthy' person, so I had to try harder, get thinner, achieve more. **Shirley**

In Western society, there are different stereotypes of the ideal body image for men and for women. The media is influential in the setting up of an image of the ideal woman as young, slim and sexually attractive.

> I was afraid of being regarded as fat, because I felt that fat women have little status in our society, are viewed as 'failures', are the butt of senseless jokes and are not seen as individuals. **Shirley**

Women in our society are generally still expected to take daily responsibility for providing food – planning meals, shopping, preparing, cooking and presenting meals. The pressures on women to be slim, dynamic, sexually attractive *and* to be a homemaker lead to conflicts about their body image and their role in life. This results in most women feeling dissatisfied with their bodies and regularly putting themselves on diets regardless of whether or not they are overweight. Dieting is rarely successful in the long term, and it does not change the size and shape of the particular body parts that are causing concern. Dieting can leave people believing they are failures – they feel they cannot even take control of their own eating and body size. This leads them to dislike themselves and their own bodies even more.

In more recent times, teenage boys have come under pressure from their peers to take care of their appearance and spend more time and money on their clothes and grooming. Boys have become much more concerned about their body image. Unlike women, men often want to *increase* their body size and muscle mass, by eating more or working out at the gym, to help them develop a 'six-pack', conform to the masculine stereotype and feel more acceptable and more powerful.

> I'd love to be bigger, I look too skinny. I'm embarrassed about my body but I can't get myself to eat so I can put weight back on. You expect men to be gladiator-like muscle men. Being thin isn't socially acceptable for men, being big and muscle-bound is. **Rhys**

Women usually want to be thinner than they are but cannot stop themselves overeating, whereas men often want to be bigger than they are but some, like Rhys, cannot get themselves to eat. Men want to develop muscle tone not flab; they are not expected to be fat, but they are under pressure to be big, powerful and muscular.

The media has always exerted a strong influence on girls, and now boys as well, to conform to particular body shapes. The current obsession of young people with taking 'selfies', and posting them on social media, leads to them constantly observing and judging their own appearance. Nowadays, children of all ages have easy access to internet pornography; and viewing this has become another pressure on them to try to achieve body shapes, including genital shapes and sizes, that are not achievable for most people. These pressures to conform to masculine and feminine stereotypes result in many women dieting, on and off, throughout their lives, and to some men trying to build up their body mass and transform their body shape.

However, only some people go on to develop eating disorders. Whether a person develops an eating disorder is the result of further individual pressures such as the eating habits within their families (particularly the mother's relationship with food and dieting), their own weight history and history of dieting, pressures to diet or body-build from peers and how they have learnt to cope with their emotions. Women still have a lower status in our society and often feel powerless in the outside world. When they have problems, they are more likely than men to turn inwards and try to control their bodies instead of dealing with the outside world. Women in high-powered jobs may turn to food as a way of coping with stress.

Childhood abuse leaves victims feeling very bad about themselves and their bodies. Many survivors block off their feelings about themselves and memories of the abuse by becoming preoccupied with their body size and their eating habits, and thus may develop an eating problem. In the next section, we look at why survivors in particular are prone to developing eating problems.

Sexual abuse and eating problems – issues in common

About 30–40 per cent of women who have eating disorders have been sexually abused as children and young people. What are the links between sexual abuse and the development of eating problems?

BODY IMAGE
As described above, eating problems usually develop in people who already have a poor body image and a history of dieting. When people are sexually abused, they learn to detest their own bodies.

> I used to hate my body because it had been used without my consent. I felt dirty. **Anthony**

Survivors associate their bodies with the physical and/or emotional pain, and the shame of what has been done to them. The poor body image of survivors makes them more likely to begin dieting or overeating as a way of trying to transform their bodies; and this can lead to the development of an eating problem.

SWALLOWING FEELINGS

After I became aware of the connection of my eating problem and the fact that I had been sexually abused as a child, I realized that at all the times in my life when I was under stress and felt unsafe and unsure of the future, I ate more and put on weight. This fact became especially clear to me after my daughter told me she had been sexually abused by a neighbour some years earlier. During that first week, while I was trying to get help for her and also trying to cope with the memories of my own abuse and the pain I felt, I reached for food almost non-stop. I felt very frightened, fearing that she would grow up with the same problems I had, and also fearing that I could not cope. I felt threatened. I so much wanted to be protected from all the pain, I wanted to feel safe. So, I ate and put on three or four pounds of weight in that one week. **Katarina**

Survivors are left with many traumatic memories and bad feelings about themselves. We all know how easy it is to reach for food when we feel bad. It doesn't take away the bad feelings but it does push them down – we swallow our bad feelings and may, briefly, feel better. Overeating can be useful at first by blocking off bad feelings and bringing a sense of relief. The bad feelings about the abuse are still there, but they become buried deep inside.

Instead, survivors are left feeling bad about breaking their diets and they feel out of control, stupid, guilty and fat. They are therefore left with bad feelings about themselves, instead of anger at their abusers or sadness about their childhoods. They often feel so bad about themselves that they reach out for more food to help them swallow their feelings again. Eating to avoid bad feelings can become such a habit that people sometimes start to binge-eat in response to any uncomfortable feeling or minor difficulty. People often reach out for chocolate when they overeat; chocolate releases endorphins that can help your mood improve. Many people with eating problems end up feeling completely numb and out of touch with their feelings. On the other hand, some survivors have feelings of guilt and shame but cannot remember anything about the abuse itself.

People who suffer from bulimia cannot cope with having unfilled or unstructured time ahead of them. They often binge-eat to distract themselves and fill the time to keep away unwanted memories, thoughts and feelings.

GUILT

Although the responsibility for sexual abuse always lies with the abuser, the victims of abuse nearly always feel guilty and blame themselves. Survivors sometimes harm themselves as a form of self-punishment for being so 'bad'. The physical pain may also help by blocking off the emotional distress. Dieting itself can be a form of self-deprivation and self-punishment.

People who are dieting inevitably overeat at times, and then feel greedy and guilty because they have broken their diet. It may be easier for them to cope with the guilt about overeating rather than the guilt about the abuse itself. Unfortunately, this leaves survivors feeling worse about *themselves*, while the real problems resulting from the sexual abuse remain unresolved. People who deliberately vomit, or take laxatives, diuretics or diet pills, are attempting to lose weight by getting rid of the calories they have just consumed, but these are also powerful ways of punishing themselves to help cope with the feelings of guilt.

SHAME

> The abuse changed my life from a very early age. I was ashamed of my body and frightened that people would be able to tell what was happening just by looking at my body. **Kate**

Many survivors feel great shame because of what has happened to them, whether they feel guilty or not. For some, dieting is a way of purifying the body and attempting to make the body perfect rather than dirty or shameful. The extreme form of this is anorexia nervosa, where women are often striving to be perfect in body and mind.

People who suffer from bulimia nervosa and deliberately vomit after eating feel great shame and disgust at their own behaviour. Deliberately vomiting, and then feeling self-disgust because you have vomited, may be a safer way for survivors to express their feelings of disgust about the abuse. Unfortunately, this means survivors then end up feeling more disgusted at themselves, instead of feeling disgusted at what the abusers did to them. For some survivors, it may be that vomiting after overeating is repeating what happened to them as children and young people when they vomited, or wanted to vomit, after being sexually abused, particularly after oral sex.

SECRECY

Common to all the eating problems is the need to eat in secret. People with eating problems will often not eat in public or will eat very little in front of other people. Their eating is mostly done in secret and may involve secret episodes of vomiting. People with bulimia nervosa are usually so ashamed of their binge-eating and vomiting that they go to great lengths to make sure no one finds out about it. Bulimia has been called the 'secret disorder', and sexual abuse and eating disorders share this theme of secrecy. Sexual abuse always occurs in secret and may be kept secret for many years.

FEELING OUT OF CONTROL

Sexual abuse is forced on to children and young people by the power and authority an adult or older child has over them. Children and young people may also feel powerless to resist because of threats, or actual physical violence, from the abuser or because they feel very confused about what is happening to them. When people are feeling powerless and out of control, the one thing they can control is their own body. Small children who are being abused often overeat, refuse to eat or wet or soil themselves (see Chapter 5). These are bodily functions that they alone can control and that adults cannot take control of.

If the feelings of powerlessness and loss of control develop as the child grows up, focusing on the body may again become a means of trying to regain some control. Some people try to control and transform their bodies by dieting and exercising. While dieting is an attempt to feel in control, the feelings of powerlessness are also expressed through losing control when bingeing and overeating. Unfortunately, the feelings of powerlessness increase when dieting does not work or when control is lost and binging results.

EATING FOR PROTECTION

Women who overeat often experience conflict in their feelings about being overweight. On a conscious level, they usually hate the idea of being fat and desperately want to become slim. However, when they explore their underlying feelings they sometimes find, to their great surprise, that they are actually terrified of being *thin*. Some survivors believe that being fat makes them unattractive to others and therefore prevents any unwanted sexual advances. For others, being fat makes them feel physically stronger, while being thin makes them feel vulnerable. Men also find it difficult to deal with feeling vulnerable, and may consciously want to get bigger and heavier to feel more powerful and more able to protect themselves.

A woman may also feel that, when she is overweight, she has more presence, power and identity because she is seen as a person rather than as a woman. Being overweight can therefore be very useful for a survivor who does not want to be seen as sexually attractive or who feels vulnerable and powerless because of the sexual abuse.

The underlying reasons for overeating vary for each individual, but being fat often has a protective function. This is why some people find they can lose weight fairly easily at first but then, as their weight drops, their hidden fears begin to surface and they start overeating again.

Concern about their bodies and eating becomes an obvious and initially useful way for survivors to deal with difficult emotions. Through dieting, bingeing and purging, survivors can express many of their feelings relating to their body image, guilt and shame. Usually, however, they end up with more bad feelings about *themselves*, instead of about the underlying problem (the sexual abuse). To overcome an eating problem, you need to start uncovering the underlying bad feelings, accepting them and expressing them.

Overcoming the problem

During the last few months I have again had a few times when I was under great stress but I have learned so much. I have learned that there is a lot more strength in me than I thought, and that no matter how difficult a situation may seem, somehow time dilutes the pain and solutions can and will be found. Instead of running away from my problems and feelings by eating I must face them and deal with them. I had a few days lately which were really difficult to cope with. But suddenly, as the problems had been solved, I realized that I ate normally during those times. No more eating non-stop, no more putting on weight. I don't need this protection any more. I can only think that this is because I feel strong enough to cope with anything the future will bring and don't want to run away any more. Nowadays I eat anything

I want to and I am gradually losing weight. The irony of the situation is that now I like my body and losing weight is totally unimportant to me. **Katarina**

To overcome an eating problem, you have to find ways of allowing the emotional issues to surface again and find more useful ways of coping with them. It is also important to look at your eating and dieting behaviour because bad habits of weight control can also lead to the development and maintenance of eating problems. If you have an established eating problem or have difficulty in regaining control of your eating, you may struggle to resolve this by yourself and would benefit from getting some professional help (see 'Sources of help' at the back of the book for details of organizations to contact for therapy, counselling and support).

STRICT DIETING

An eating problem rarely develops without a history of strict dieting. People put themselves on diets in order to lose weight (often when they are not even overweight to start with), but strict dieting rarely helps anyone lose weight in the long term. In fact, repeated dieting slows the metabolic rate (the speed at which the body burns up calories). After a return to normal eating, a slower metabolic rate can cause weight to be gained a lot more quickly, so people who diet often end up heavier than they were before they started dieting – it may be that only 5 per cent of people who diet are able to maintain the weight loss.

When people are dieting, they are trying to control their bodies and they stop listening to physiological signals. They try to ignore the signals telling them they are hungry and that their bodies need food. This self-starvation acts as a threat to the body's survival and leads to a preoccupation with food. If they break the self-imposed diet by eating something 'bad' (for example, high-calorie food), they feel they have lost control. They often then overeat as a way of coping with feeling out of control. Strict dieting not only makes people fatter but can also lead on to binge-eating or overeating. The first step in overcoming an eating problem is to *stop strict dieting for ever*. This does not mean you cannot try to lose weight if you need to. A more practical way of losing weight is described later in this chapter.

EXPLORING YOUR FEELINGS ABOUT YOUR BODY SIZE
People with eating problems use eating, or not eating, and pre-occupation with their body shape, as a way of coping with their emotions. To stabilize your weight at a reasonable level and develop a healthy relationship with your body and food, you need to uncover the feelings you are hiding from and find more useful ways of working with them.

Some women have an underlying, unconscious, fear of becoming fat or fatter. Exploring your feelings about your weight often helps you see that being fat may also feel useful to you in some way. It may make you feel protected and safe, sexually unattractive or more powerful. It is clearly very difficult for you to regain control of your eating, or lose weight, if you have underlying fears about becoming slim.

BINGE-EATING
Binge-eating is usually triggered by an unpleasant event, stress, bad feelings or memories.

> My weight fluctuates between 10 and 13 stone. I don't eat very often. Sometimes I don't eat for a week, I just drink tea. Then something makes me feel bad and I binge on chocolates and chocolate biscuits. **Rhys**

Often the person is feeling deprived of love, safety or comfort. They want or feel 'something' but don't know what this 'something' is. They are invariably already dieting or restricting their food intake and are feeling hungry, so they reach out for food. You can use your urge to binge-eat, or urge to eat when you are not hungry, as a way of finding out what you really want or what feelings you are avoiding.

Exercise: What do you really want?

1 Next time you feel you are going to binge, try delaying the binge for 10 minutes. If you find this difficult, try 5 minutes or 1 minute.
2 Do something *for yourself* in this 10 minutes instead of binge-eating – for example, have a bath, read a magazine, go on social media, phone a friend, do a mindfulness meditation or yoga, or go for a run. Think of things you enjoy doing that are free or

cheap, last 10 to 20 minutes and are nothing to do with food. Write these treats down (on paper or on the notes page of your phone); it helps to write a list of these non-food treats when you are in a good mood and not hungry. Instead of binge-eating, give yourself one of your treats. Binge afterwards if you really have to.

3 The first step is to learn to delay the binge, as above. Learning that you can delay a binge may also help you feel more in control.

4 Once you can delay binge-eating for 10 minutes by replacing it with treats as above, the next step is to use this 10-minute delay to sit quietly, relax and think 'What do I really want? What am I really feeling?' This exercise is a way for you to find out what triggers off a binge and to discover what you really want and feel.

5 If feelings like guilt, shame and so on surface, you can work on them by using the ideas from the other chapters in this book, or just experience the emotions. If you feel sad because you cannot get what you want immediately, you may want to express this by crying or just feeling sad. It is better to cry because you are sad than to eat because you are sad.

6 Learn to eat whatever you want to, *if you really want it*. Don't eat if you find that you are actually feeling sad, angry or hurt rather than hungry.

7 When you begin to take control of binge-eating, you may initially feel more depressed as your buried problems begin to surface; but now you have the opportunity to deal with the issues directly, instead of thinking about food and worrying about your weight. You may need to get some professional help with this.

PURGING

After binge-eating, many people learn to purge themselves by making themselves vomit up all the food they have eaten, or by taking large quantities of laxatives, diuretics or diet pills. These are all attempts to get rid of the calories just consumed and therefore avoid becoming fat. All these ways of purging are physically very dangerous. There are many unpleasant and medically dangerous side effects of purging, including damage to the teeth and gums, throat haemorrhages and electrolyte disturbances (which can lead to epilepsy, kidney failure and other very serious conditions).

None of these methods of purging eliminates all the calories. Laxatives only prevent a very small proportion of the calories from being absorbed. However many times you vomit, you will still only prevent a proportion of the calories from being absorbed. Some people with eating problems exercise excessively instead of purging – the ideas below can help you understand and control the level of exercise you take.

Try using the same technique (as above) to control your purging as you do to understand your binge-eating; that is, create a delay before you purge or engage in excessive exercise and use this time to reflect and find out *why* you are doing it. Perhaps you will discover that purging (which is painful and dangerous) is a way of punishing yourself, or of indirectly expressing your anger or other bad feelings.

> Controlling my weight by vomiting was a way of coping with the hatred I felt towards myself; and it was a secret expression of the anger I felt inside myself but was too afraid to direct at the real causes of my anger. I could literally swallow my anger and pain by eating, then purge myself of it. **Shirley**

Most people who stop binge-eating also stop purging. If you do not stop purging, try to use the technique described above or seek professional help.

HOW TO LOSE WEIGHT

If you feel that you have explored and worked through your feelings about your weight and you are *realistically* overweight, you may want to try to lose some weight. It is obviously very difficult to lose weight before you have dealt with any fears about being slim and any other underlying disturbing emotions. The method below will not work unless you have overcome these fears. If you have been dieting on and off for years, you may find it difficult to lose weight because your metabolism may have slowed down.

- Stop strict dieting. Try to eat three meals a day, however small.
- Aim to lose 1 or 2 pounds a week *maximum*. If you lose more than this, it will be water, not fat, that you are losing; and the weight loss will be difficult to maintain.
- One pound of fat is equivalent to about 3,500 calories; so to lose

1 pound of fat per week, you need to cut 3,500 calories per week (or 500 calories per day) from your usual calorie intake.

- Aim to cut about 250 calories a day *only* off your normal eating, by cutting down on your fat and sugar intake. Try to replace fatty food and junk food with wholefood. Junk food contains many calories but does not provide the nutrients your body needs, so you very quickly become hungry again after you have eaten it. Eating healthy foods will make you feel better as well as assisting you in controlling your weight.
- Burn off the other 250 calories a day by doing some exercise. Exercise not only burns off calories but can increase your metabolic rate, so you will burn off more calories whatever you are doing. If you try to lose weight without doing exercise, you will lose water and lean tissue (muscle) instead of the fat you want to lose. Useful exercise can be going for a brisk walk, gardening or cleaning – it doesn't have to be going to the gym.

Remember that strict dieting is very unlikely to help you lose weight and keep the weight off. You may actually end up heavier, feeling deprived and thinking about food all the time. You will also be more likely to overeat whenever you do break your diet.

BODY IMAGE

Most of my problems have gone. What has taken me longer is to accept that it is possible for a man to look at me without feeling repulsion. My poor body image and my eating problem have been with me for so long that they will take longer to leave me. **Katarina**

Disliking your body can distort your own perception of your body so that it appears to you to be bigger and fatter than it actually is. You really can see yourself as fat, when objectively you may be normal weight or even thin. Men may see their bodies as too thin and not masculine or 'normal' enough.

I think I was too busy trying to look normal, so no one would discover my secret. I did get obsessional about my body and went to the gym excessively. **Luke**

It is possible to change your perception of your own body but it takes a lot of practice over a period of time. You have spent many years building a distorted body image, so it will take time to see it accurately again.

Exercise: Mirror work
When most women look in a full-length mirror, they focus on the part of their bodies that they dislike the most – their stomachs, hips, breasts and so on. This distorts the way they see themselves. Men may also focus on the parts of their bodies they dislike – their chests, legs, arms, stomach and so on. Try looking in a full-length mirror when naked. What parts do you focus on? If you hate your thighs because you think they are too big, focusing on them makes them appear even bigger *to you*. If you feel your chest is narrow and puny, focusing on it will make it appear even smaller *to you*. Try to look at *the whole* of your body. Try not to judge it, just look at it. Try to accept and like yourself, saying, 'This is my body.' Do this exercise twice a day when you are getting dressed and undressed.

Summary

Many women dislike their own bodies and are preoccupied with food and body image. Men and boys are also experiencing a lot of media and peer pressure about their body image and how they are supposed to look. Images and articles on the internet put even more pressure on boys and girls to achieve an impossible 'perfect' body shape. Strict dieting and restricting food are ways of trying to transform the body but rarely lead to permanent weight loss or the desired body shape, and usually leave people fatter and feeling even less in control of their lives than before. Some people then go on to develop more serious problems such as binge-eating and bulimia nervosa.

Many survivors develop difficulties around eating as a way of coping with their emotional problems. Both people with eating problems and survivors of sexual abuse have feelings of dislike or disgust towards their own bodies. They also share feelings of guilt, shame, low self-worth and feeling out of control. Difficulties around eating may result in survivors experiencing a temporary relief from their distress about the abuse as their memories and bad feelings resulting from the abuse become buried. In the long term, the eating problems can lead to medical complications and a further lowering of self-esteem.

To overcome an eating problem, it is necessary to allow the underlying memories and feelings to surface so that they can be processed and dealt with. One way of doing this is to explore what you are thinking and feeling when you reach out for food. It is also important to change your behaviours around food – for example, binge-eating, purging or excessive exercising. In order to do this, it is important that you stop strict dieting. As you grow to understand and accept yourself, you will probably find you can also learn to respect and accept your own body.

> Sharing the pain with other women helped me to find better ways of coping. As the wounds caused by the abuse began to heal, as I began to see myself as a whole person, where the good in me began to feel as real as the bad things I had found in myself, I no longer saw myself as being fat. I am free of the bulimia because I am free of the abuse, free of the guilt, free of the hate, and I am free to find in myself the person that I want to be, not the person I am afraid to be. **Shirley**

What to do next

1 Follow the suggestions and exercises described above, to help you stop dieting and to begin to overcome your eating and body image problems.
2 Seek professional help if you have a serious eating disorder or have difficulty in gaining control of your eating or dieting. See 'Sources of help' at the back of this book.
3 Try not to deprive yourself (by dieting or ignoring your own needs or feelings). Spend time on yourself and your own needs.

A helpful resource for young people concerned about their eating behaviour can found at:

<https://youngminds.org.uk/media/1517/youngminds-eating-problems-yp.pdf>.

11

Sex and sexuality

Many adult survivors of childhood sexual abuse experience difficulties with sex and relationships as a result of their inappropriate and usually disturbing introduction to sexual matters. For children and young people who are not sexually abused, sexuality is a developing process. They gradually become aware of, and explore, their own bodies, their own sexuality and their relationships with other people. Knowledge and experience develop slowly, giving the child time to adjust at each stage. Sexual experiences should be associated with good feelings and with pleasure and relaxation. Even though teenagers often pressurize each other about relationships, they can still make their own choices about who they want to develop sexual relationships with and how far to go. Children who are sexually abused have no control over this process and are thus prevented from developing their knowledge and sexual experience at their own pace.

We discussed the process of 'traumatic sexualization' in Chapter 2. When children and young people are sexually abused, they are introduced to sexual acts that are not appropriate to their age or level of development, and this can be very confusing for them.

> When I got out of the bath, my uncle took the towel and started rubbing me all over my body. He began touching my penis and he kept asking me if I liked what he was doing. The next thing I was on the floor and I felt something wet on my backside, I now know it was Vaseline. He penetrated me and I cried out telling him to stop it, it was hurting me that much. When he stopped, I was crying my eyes out. He told me every little boy and girl cry the first time but now I wasn't a virgin because he had broken me in. He said when you grow up you will know how to do sex. I just couldn't understand what was happening. **Anthony**

Children and young people may be forced, or manipulated, into submitting to sexual acts or doing things they do not want to do.

Abusers often punish children who try to object to the abuse, or give presents, money or affection if they submit to sexual acts. Young people learn that sex can be exchanged for rewards, and some continue to use sex in this way in adult life. The sexual abuse is often confusing, frightening or physically painful, so sex becomes associated with negative feelings: fear, shame, tension and dirtiness. The abuse may also be associated with good feelings, with affection, physical pleasure and orgasms. This can leave the child or teenager feeling even more confused.

> He rubbed my clitoris with his finger until I had an orgasm. It was very confusing because while I liked the feelings it produced, I hated it because it was him who made it happen. My own body had now betrayed me. **Sandra**

Even if the abuse involves some pleasant physical sensations, children are still subjected to sexual experiences they have not chosen or that are too advanced for their age, and with inappropriate people such as family members, adults or older children. Children and young people do not have any control over the situation. They are not able to make choices about their sexual experiences, or to develop sexually at their own pace with their peers. Their experiences are very different from those of young people who have not been sexually abused.

This process of traumatic sexualization leads to a variety of sexual problems in the adult survivor. Not all survivors experience sexual problems, but many women with sexual problems have been sexually abused.

This chapter looks at some of the sexual problems experienced by survivors, and suggests ways of understanding and overcoming these difficulties. The chapter is for people of any sex or gender, sexual orientation and sexual identity, and for people with or without partners. It is for anyone who is interested in understanding more about their sexual feelings and learning to be more comfortable about sexual matters, as well as for people with specific sexual difficulties.

Ingrid, in her story below, describes the sexual difficulties she experienced through her teenage and adult life as a result of being abused as a child.

Ingrid's story

I was sexually abused from when I was 4 years old. In the years that followed as I grew into the age of harmless dates with boys, I guessed that my feelings and attitudes were not the same as those of my friends. I had no way of relating to boys. My mother wanted to protect me and did not allow me to talk to or play with the boys in our neighbourhood. The only boy I knew was my brother and he abused me. When my friends started to go out with boys and in giggles and whispers talked about kissing in doorways, I did not understand them. As they talked I could almost feel my brother forcing his tongue down my throat and felt repulsion and disgust. My friends all seemed happy and excited. I felt an outsider.

By the time I was sexually involved with a man at the age of 16, I knew that my emotions were crippled, my feelings distorted. I looked at other girls and wondered why I could not be like them. I fell in love as totally as my friends, but when it came to kissing, touching and finally sex, I froze and lost all feelings. I felt numb, paralysed, trapped. I agreed to sex more out of gratitude than desire and because I didn't know how to say 'No'. He was the first man who wanted me, the first who did not get bored with me after 2 or 3 weeks because I was so quiet, and he really seemed to like me. So when I became pregnant when I was 17, we got married.

At first I thought I was too young to like sex. I knew something was not right with the way I hated any physical contact. Maybe the problems would not have grown as large if he had been a more patient and understanding man. He knew about the abuse but did not care much. But sex was very important to him. It was never love-making, only sex. There was never any love-play involved. As I was cooking dinner, he pulled me away into the bedroom, with a wide grin pulled down my pants and had intercourse. At other times he came from behind when I was busy with something and suddenly masturbated all over me. But when I had time I was expected to be always ready and always willing to satisfy him. He wanted me to have an insatiable sexual appetite and initiate sex several times a day. To please him I tried to be like that but sometimes the disgust with my own behaviour, the repulsion with the way he wanted sex was so great I would rather let him beat me. I felt sexually abused all through my marriage.

The disgust I felt against my own abuser and what he did to me turned inwards and I felt disgust with myself.

I hated it. I felt as if I was degrading myself. I felt dirty. I felt humiliated, especially when I tried my hardest to please him in bed and, during intercourse, he told me that all my friends and my brother's wife were better in bed than I was. I never learned what a loving touch could be like. He never stroked me, never caressed me, never tried to arouse me. My husband was abusive, unfaithful and humiliated me. Finally when he tried to persuade me to become a prostitute, I had enough and left him. Maybe it was the sexual abuse that led me to get involved with him in the first place. Maybe it was because of the abuse that I stayed with him for 7 years.

After my divorce, I always had problems saying 'No'. I did not want sex but I had been programmed from early childhood right through the years of marriage to be submissive so that I just could not refuse. I did not think anybody could like me for what I was. I imagined my only value was to be used. I went through a period of sleeping with a number of men. I couldn't say 'No' and I was searching, without success, for some good feelings in sex, the way my friends felt, and the way it was portrayed, in gentle love-making scenes in films and books. I did not find it.

For years during my first marriage and after the divorce I kept wishing I could be a lesbian or nun so I would never have to be touched by a man again. They seemed the only acceptable reasons to refuse sexual advances. I met my second husband when I was 27. He was friendly to me and did not ask for sex. I was sure he would not physically or sexually abuse me. During my 14 years of marriage to him we rarely had sex, and when we did I blocked off any feelings of pleasure. Sometimes a touch felt nice, but as soon as I recognized it was pleasure I felt, it was like running into a brick wall. I consciously refused to enjoy any touch. Most of the time I could cope with the physical side of my marriage. But at times he behaved in a way that made me, once again, see myself as dirty. At times like those I could feel myself choking with disgust, as if somebody was strangling me and I could not breathe. All I wanted to do then was to run away, but I had not learnt to say 'No' or to express dislike for certain behaviour. And so all too often as soon as my husband turned towards me I froze and inside me the abused child that was still present screamed with sheer terror. After a few years I learned to develop an asthma attack as soon as my husband followed me into the bedroom or as soon as I thought he wanted sex. I knew that I was bringing the attack on myself through my own will. A whole range of sudden symptoms like urticaria [hives] and hot flushes, and so on gave me time to delay and often stopped any attempt at intimacy. At first, we used to joke that I was allergic to him, although I knew why I felt ill.

Until I married my second husband I had felt disgust with sex, in later years it turned into indifference. During therapy, I gradually began to realize that I could allow myself to feel sexual pleasure without feeling disgusted and dirty. Now my sexual problems have gone and I regret bitterly the wasted years of being unable to enjoy intimacy when it was offered. **Ingrid**

Sexual problems

Box 8 shows some of the physical and sexual difficulties that are often experienced by teenage and adult survivors of sexual abuse. Survivors may experience different types of sexual problems at different times in their lives. Some of them are discussed below.

AVOIDING PHYSICAL CONTACT AND RELATIONSHIPS
Some survivors dislike all forms of physical contact and avoid any touch or closeness such as friendly hugs, handshakes or even sitting next to someone. Many survivors find the idea of sexual contact especially unpleasant, frightening or disturbing and may therefore avoid relationships. This often begins when the survivor is a teenager.

When my girlfriends at school were experimenting with boys I shied away. **Jocelyn**

I didn't like boyfriends or being on my own with men. I used to spend a lot of time in my bedroom on my own. **Polly**

Avoiding relationships adds to a teenage survivor's feelings of isolation and of being different from other people. Anita recalls being teased at school for not having boyfriends and for being sexually inexperienced. These problems may gradually disappear as a teenage survivor reaches adulthood and manages to form relationships and deal with physical contact. However, some survivors carry the fear of physical contact into adulthood and avoid relationships altogether.

Box 8 Sexual difficulties

- Dislike of touching or looking at oneself.
- Dislike or avoidance of relationships.
- Dislike or avoidance of physical contact.
- Dislike or avoidance of sexual contact.
- Dislike or avoidance of certain sexual activities.
- Lack of physical pleasure in sex.
- Dissociating or switching off during sex.
- Flashbacks during sex.
- Inability to have an orgasm.
- Vaginismus (tightening spasms of the vaginal muscles).
- Not being able to say 'No' to sex.
- Having sex indiscriminately.
- Prostitution.
- Aggressive sexual behaviour.
- Disturbing sexual fantasies.
- Sexual pleasure linked to pain.
- Feeling guilty about sex.
- Thinking sex is dirty or disgusting.
- Confusion about sexual orientation (heterosexual/homosexual).
- Lack of accurate sexual knowledge.
- Sexualizing relationships and situations.
- Obsession with sex.
- Obsession with masturbating.

INDISCRIMINATE SEX

In contrast, many survivors report that they have gone through a phase of having indiscriminate sex with many different people. This may start at an early age or follow a period of avoiding relationships and physical contact.

Jocelyn shied away from boys as a young teenager but went through a period of indiscriminate sexual activity with many men in her late teens and early twenties.

> When I did eventually sleep with someone I became promiscuous. Sex didn't really mean anything. My feelings didn't enter into it. I was living a role. **Jocelyn**

Like Jocelyn, many survivors have learnt as children and young people to separate their emotions from their sexual activities. As adults, sex may become a meaningless activity. Many survivors feel that it doesn't matter what happens to them or their bodies any more. As a teenager, finding someone to have sex with and staying out at night may also be a way of avoiding going home to the abuser.

Many survivors feel unable to say 'No' to sex or feel that they have no choice and no control over their bodies.

> I'm afraid of saying 'No' to sexual advances. Often, I initiate them in order to be in control of the situation and then end up getting a bad reputation. **Paula**

Sexually abused children learn that they cannot say 'No' to sex; they have no choice. Children and young people often believe that they were responsible for the sexual abuse because they think they caused the abuser to become sexually excited. As adults, survivors may still believe that they are responsible for other people becoming sexually aroused and therefore feel they must satisfy them.

> I have been in situations where, when I look back, I could have said 'No' to sex but I have felt unable to say 'No'. I often felt that I had led the other person on in some way. I did not realize that men should be in control of their own bodies. I did not want to be called a 'cock teaser'. My stepfather called me a 'bitch on heat' when I was 13 because I was out with a few friends who just happened to be boys. Perhaps I believed him. **Jane**

Survivors who find little pleasure in sex, or experience sexual problems, may try to find a solution to these difficulties by having sex with many different people. For some survivors, sex is an attempt to get close to someone and receive some comfort, although they often end up feeling dissatisfied or even more lonely, disgusted and ashamed.

> I was desperate for someone to like me, desperate for some feeling of tenderness, caring, comfort and closeness. I remember days when I stood at the window, alone in my flat, looking out and waiting. I was so lonely that I would have taken anybody, and I mean anybody, as lover or friend, just to know someone cared. I would have sold my soul to the devil for somebody to put his arms around me with genuine feelings of liking me. There were a few men I only knew one evening before we had sex. I searched for love and closeness, but the morning after when I woke up

the only feeling I had was of desperation, shame, guilt and a terrible emptiness. After a few months of searching for friendship and love I withdrew. I did not go out any more and so did not get into contact with men any more who were interested only in satisfying their sexual desire. The few moments of tenderness and holding were not worth the loneliness and the bad feelings afterwards. **Katarina**

For some survivors, indiscriminate and unsatisfactory sex becomes a pattern they continue throughout their adult life. Many survivors, however, opt for one-to-one relationships or revert back to avoiding relationships. They often feel ashamed of what they describe as their 'promiscuous phase'. Fiona has come to understand that picking up men was a reaction to her loneliness and fear and is now able to accept herself without judgement:

I felt lonely most of my childhood but when I got to 17 and my mother left home, I was extremely lonely. I'd go with men at night who I met in pubs and night clubs. I never intended to have sex with them, I just wanted to be with someone. I hated going home alone. The house was so empty, everywhere was so empty. I was looking desperately for someone to care. When I did find the odd man who cared for me, I rejected him. I couldn't accept love so I just got hurt time after time with the ones who just wanted one thing. I'd sleep most of the day till it was time to go to the pub. Some nights I'd sit at the bottom of our estate hoping to find someone to talk to. The feeling as I sat there was as if I was chained to that place and I was crying out for someone to come and take me away. It was a big empty dark world out there but I'd pray every night that someone (Mr Right) would come for me and I could love him and he'd love me. Some nights if I'd been to a night club and hadn't 'pulled', I'd walk home alone feeling so desperate. Then my desperation would turn to anger. I would want to cry but couldn't. My throat would feel so tight, I could hardly swallow so I would get angrier, and try harder to cry but couldn't. I would think of throwing myself under a car but I didn't have the guts. I'd finally get home, pig myself with food, smoke a cig and sleep the clock around.

On the other hand, if I did 'pull' it usually ended up with them having sex with me. To them I was just another screw. I'd go home, usually the next day, feeling more depressed, and cry and feel ashamed. I'd usually fall in love with that kind (well, I thought it was love) and end up feeling hurt and used when they didn't speak to me the next time I saw them. There seemed to be no hope for me.

I'm free now, and with writing this for the first time I've realized that. I realize how bad I felt growing up and I can see how I've carried a lot of emotions and hurt into my adult life. I also know now that I wasn't a slag at 17 years old. I was an empty, lonely, frightened young girl who had never loved or been loved. The nearest to love I got was being sexually abused time and time again, but now I'm learning to love. **Fiona**

Survivors who go through periods of having sex with lots of people may see sex as a meaningless activity, or be desperately trying to seek some affection and closeness, or feel unable to say 'No' to sex.

AVOIDING OR DISLIKING SEX

Many survivors dislike sex or find it disgusting or boring. Survivors often marry or live with a partner, but they may still dislike sex and try to avoid it whenever possible. Some survivors marry but do not consummate their marriages. Others live with people who are not particularly interested in sex and therefore make few sexual demands. Ingrid chose a sexually undemanding man as her second husband. Many survivors find excuses for not having sex or bring on physical symptoms to avoid sex: Anita avoided sex throughout her pregnancy; Ingrid developed rashes and had asthma attacks.

However, many survivors do have sex, even though they dislike it or do not get pleasure from it. Sometimes this is done for their partners' sake or because they feel they have no choice. Some women may feel it is their duty to have sex, however much they dislike it. Men can also feel under pressure to perform and that they 'should' want to have sex whenever there is an opportunity.

My first husband didn't understand why I had never played the field, so to speak. My first sexual experience, besides my father, was my first husband and then I never relaxed. I was always uptight and ended up crying most times. That marriage ended in divorce. **Pam**

Some survivors lie passively and let their partner have sex with them without participating. Often they are repeating what happened when they were being abused. Some survivors realize they can still dissociate or switch off during sex, just like they did as children. They may dislike sex or have no interest in sex but continue to switch off and have sex, perhaps because they feel they have no choice, or they want to please their partners, or they want to appear 'normal'.

Dislike of sex is usually a result of the bad feelings that became associated with sex during the abuse. Feelings of fear, tension, guilt and shame can prevent survivors from experiencing any sexual pleasure. Guilt about having sex, or getting pleasure from sex, can cause survivors to block out good feelings during sex or touching, leaving them feeling dissatisfied or disgusted.

For some survivors, there is no pleasure in sex, for others the pleasurable feelings may come and go.

TURN-OFFS

During sexual activity, survivors may suddenly 'turn off' sexually or feel frightened, angry or disgusted. This often happens because something (a word, a smell, a certain type of touch, or sexual position) has triggered off memories of the abuse.

This is not always a conscious process; they may simply feel bad or lose interest in sex without realizing why. The trigger may make the survivor dissociate or cut off as they did during the abuse. Survivors often dislike certain sexual activities because they happened during the abuse (for example, oral sex) and may, as a result, feel such behaviour is perverted and disgusting. Some survivors recognize that their present feelings are connected with the abuse and that these activities are unpleasant reminders of what happened in the past.

> A lot of the things my husband does to me would be considered natural behaviour but to me they are sickening memories of my childhood abuse. **Gail**

Others may not yet have made the link between their childhood abuse and adult feelings.

Triggers that can cause survivors to turn off or start to feel bad include:

- words – breasts, father, cock;
- phrases – 'I love you', 'You like this, don't you?';
- smells – tobacco, alcohol, aftershave, perfume, engine oil;
- touches – stroking the face, grabbing the legs;

- positions – 'doggy' style;
- behaviours – oral sex, masturbation;
- clothes – jeans, dressing gown;
- others – pubic hair, false teeth, glazed eyes.

TURN-ONS

Some survivors are concerned about the kinds of things that 'turn them on' or increase their sexual arousal. They may be turned on by memories of the abuse or by objects or situations associated with the abuse. They may fantasize about the abuse or the abuser, while masturbating. Other people are aroused by behaviours that occurred during the abuse and feel driven to re-enact aspects of the abuse, either alone or with a partner. Some survivors may be horrified to find they are sexually aroused by children of a certain age, even though they know they would never act on it.

Survivors who respond sexually to people or things associated with the abuse usually feel very ashamed and guilty about this. Although it can be disturbing to become aroused by things associated with the abuse, it is a very common reaction and does not mean that you were responsible for the abuse or wanted it. It can be difficult to control what we are sexually aroused by, but we can learn to control how we act on these feelings. If you are disturbed by the things you are sexually aroused by, you might find it helpful to see a therapist.

Please get some help if you are sexually aroused by children and are planning, or fantasizing, about making sexual contact with a child (even if you believe you would not act on it). **You should seek help immediately if you are acting out, or have acted out, abuse with a child. Contact Stop it Now! (at: <www.stopitnow. org.uk>) in confidence.**

FLASHBACKS

During flashbacks, the survivor experiences a vivid memory of the abuse, so vivid that it feels like he or she is reliving the abuse. Flashbacks commonly occur during sex, but they can occur in any situation that reminds the survivor of the past abuse. A survivor may feel like a child again and see his or her partner as the abuser. This can be a terrifying experience. Some survivors hit out at their partners during flashbacks, believing them to be the abuser.

The kinds of triggers, listed above, that cause survivors to turn off or feel bad during sex can also cause flashbacks to occur. Smells in particular can be powerful triggers for flashbacks. However, *anything* can trigger a flashback. What causes a flashback to occur for an individual survivor will depend on his or her particular experiences.

> I have flashbacks. My husband once said he liked something I was doing to him and to carry on. I felt sick, these words triggered something off – the abuser was making me do something to him because he enjoyed it. **Jocelyn**

Partners may have no idea what is happening when a survivor has a flashback. They may also have little understanding of why survivors suddenly turn off during sex or start to feel bad. This can cause major difficulties in relationships and leave both the survivor and his or her partner feeling confused, frightened, upset, angry or rejected.

Flashbacks usually occur because being sexually abused is a traumatic event. Some incidents during the abuse were so horrific for the young person that his or her brain was overwhelmed and could not process what was happening; the information about the incident then remains unaltered in the brain as if it is still in the present time. A reminder of the incident can trigger off the neural circuits where the incident is held, and this is experienced by the survivor as if the terrifying incident is happening again now.

SEXUAL ORIENTATION

> I'm not gay but I hate myself because I was forced to perform gay acts. It makes it even worse that I had an erection when it was happening. I won't ever trust another man as long as I live. **Graham**

It is natural for children and young people to respond to stimulation of their genitals, whatever the sex of the abuser. Responding like this is a physical reaction and is unrelated to whether the child is heterosexual, homosexual or bisexual, but it may confuse a developing child who is unsure about what is happening and about his or her own response to the physical stimulation:

> My sexuality was deeply affected; for many years I thought I was homosexual and that it was just a matter of time before I 'came

out'. What 11-year-old boy wouldn't react the way I did when his penis was touched? I thought that made me homosexual. Yet this didn't feel right, it wasn't what I wanted although I would fantasize about men. My mother taught me that homosexuality was such a crime but now I know it doesn't matter a toss what my sexuality is. **Luke**

Luke now believes he is heterosexual but had felt confused because he had responded sexually to his male abuser's touch and had had sexual fantasies about men. Some male survivors who were abused by men have sex with as many women as possible in an attempt to cover up their worries about their own sexual orientation. There is nothing wrong or unnatural about being attracted to same-sex partners, although some people still find this difficult to accept in themselves and others. The most important thing is feeling comfortable with your choice of partner and with yourself. Being sexually abused is highly unlikely to change anyone's sexual orientation or sexual identity, but it does add to the confusion of young people who are already struggling to cope with growing up and exploring their own sexual development.

LACK OF SEXUAL KNOWLEDGE

Despite having many unwanted sexual experiences from a very early age, some survivors have very limited sexual knowledge or understanding. They may have been too young to understand what was happening during the abuse or they may have closed their minds to what was happening. Children and young people who have been sexually abused often do not show the usual curiosity about sexual matters or want to experiment like other teenagers. They may switch off in sex education lessons, and avoid any information or discussion about sex in magazines, books, TV programmes or teenage chat, on the internet or social media.

> When my teenage friends talked about sex, I either pretended I was in a hurry, or I deliberately concentrated on something different, so as not to hear anything they said. As an adult woman I wanted no knowledge of sex. It was disgusting, repulsive, humiliating. I knew all I needed to know for my purposes, that was how to bring the man to a climax as quickly as possible to get it over and done with. I wanted no further knowledge of sex. **Katarina**

Subjects that are met with embarrassed giggles by other children can be traumatic reminders of abuse for an abused child. This situation leaves many survivors in ignorance of basic knowledge about the make-up of men's and women's bodies, 'normal' sexual behaviour, contraception, sexual health and sexual diseases, pregnancy and childbirth. Many adult survivors continue to avoid matters concerning sex or sexual anatomy, and may even avoid looking at their own bodies.

> I was in my early twenties when I looked at my vagina for the first time. I did not know what it was supposed to look like, but felt sure it was deformed somehow. I immediately made an appointment with my gynaecologist who assured me I was perfectly normal. **Katarina**

Lack of accurate knowledge about sex means that survivors often do not know what would be considered 'normal' or 'abnormal' sexual behaviour and do not know how to tackle any problems that may arise.

PREOCCUPATION WITH SEX OR PARTICULAR SEXUAL PRACTICES

Some survivors appear to be preoccupied with sex. They tell sexual jokes, bring sex into every conversation and see sex in all sorts of situations. For some survivors, this is a conscious 'front' put on in order to cover up their own ignorance, insecurity and anxiety about sexual matters. Others become preoccupied with sex because so much of their childhood has been connected with sexual matters and this is how they have learnt to view the world.

Some survivors feel compelled to keep having sex or to masturbate again and again. This may be a sign of distress or else it can be a way of distracting themselves from thoughts and feelings about the abuse.

Survivors may find themselves only able to gain pleasure from particular sexual practices – for example, using certain objects, being tied up, having pain inflicted on them or inflicting pain. This often reflects activities they had to participate in during their abuse. In this way, adult survivors 'act out' their abuse through their own sexual behaviour.

PROSTITUTION

Sexual abuse can leave survivors feeling that it doesn't matter what happens to their bodies, and seeing sex as something that can be exchanged for money or goods. Survivors may therefore see prostitution as a means of supporting themselves when they have no other way of earning money.

Studies have found that many prostitutes (60 to 85 per cent) were sexually abused as children and young people. Prostitution may be one of the few ways to get access to money for teenagers who have run away from home to escape the abuse, or for survivors who have lost out on their education, have small children to support or are in abusive relationships. Some survivors, both male and female, feel that prostitution is a way of taking back control and getting even, by making men pay for services they were forced to give as a child. Sadly, some survivors just do not care what happens to them. Survivors may be forced into prostitution by abusive partners or family members.

Some may have been used as child prostitutes when they were young by their abusers, who would pass them on to other perpetrators. Graham's mother sexually abused him and sold him for the use of a paedophile network at the weekends.

Overcoming the problems

You may find yourself becoming less negative about sex as you work your way through this book and begin to feel less guilty and ashamed about what has happened. Try to keep in mind that it isn't sex that's painful and frightening, but being sexually abused – your body was assaulted and your feelings were disregarded. A consensual adult sexual relationship can result in pleasurable sexual feelings, and sexual experiences alone, or with a partner, can be loving and enjoyable.

> As I begin to love myself and my body I have also discovered that to have sex with someone I love deeply is the highest expression of joy, a celebration of being alive. My hunger for knowledge about my own body and that of my partner is insatiable. A whole new world is opening up for me. Now a kiss can move the earth and a touch takes away all gravity and makes me feel as if I can fly. **Ingrid**

Sexual problems cannot be dealt with in isolation. They are closely bound up with a person's physical and emotional state of health, relationship with their partner, feelings of self-worth, body image, sexual knowledge and the ideas they have about what sex should and should not involve.

PHYSICAL AND EMOTIONAL HEALTH

When people are anxious and depressed, they often lose their interest and enjoyment in sex. If you are feeling distressed, it may be better to work through some of the other chapters in this book or seek help with your emotional problems before tackling your sexual problems directly. It is difficult to enjoy sex if you are depressed, anxious, angry or tense. Give yourself time to feel better emotionally before dealing with this area.

The same applies to physical health. Physical injury, illness, poor health or tiredness can all lead to disinterest in, or aversion to, sex. Taking certain medication can also affect your interest in sex. Wait until you are feeling more physically healthy before tackling your sexual difficulties.

RELATIONSHIPS

Sexual problems are often associated with tension, anger, misunderstanding and lack of communication between partners. There is little hope of having a good sexual relationship with a partner if your relationship in general is not very good. It may be that you are angry with your partner for something he or she has done or not done. Maybe you feel hurt, neglected or just bored. This needs to be dealt with first before you can deal with the sexual problems. Talking about how you are feeling with your partner instead of bottling up bad feelings is a useful start. Confidence-building or assertion training can help with this.

Change becomes possible once you start to communicate more openly. You may have chosen a partner that you do not feel sexually attracted to because he or she seemed 'safe' and undemanding, or because you accepted the first person who wanted you. You may feel so indebted to your partner just for being with you that you feel you need to pay him or her back with sex. Sex can become a focus for many other problems. Sometimes sex turns into a power struggle between partners: not having sex or having sex can become a way of punishing the other person or a way of taking control.

You may need to get outside help or sort out problems in your relationship. A third party can often see more clearly what is going on in a relationship. Your local branch of Relate will probably be able to help. Counselling can help partners understand each other better and strengthen their relationship. It can also give people the courage to leave relationships that are not good for them. Survivors are more likely to become involved in abusive relationships as adults, as we discussed in Chapter 2, and as some of the survivors' stories in this book have already illustrated.

NO PARTNER
You may not have a partner at the moment, or may have never had a partner. Don't be put off by our references to relationships or partners; these exercises are for you too. Having time and space free from a relationship can be useful for exploring your sexuality, expanding your knowledge and understanding, and feeling more comfortable with your body. If you wish to form a relationship but have been held back by your fear, anxiety or anger, working through these exercises can help you begin to understand these feelings and become more relaxed and open to other people.

Exercise: Obstacles to forming a sexual relationship
Write down all the things that you feel are holding you back from having a relationship with someone else. Include any fears and anxieties about being close to someone and trusting them, and any fears about the sexual side of a relationship.

MYTHS AND MESSAGES
The first step in exploring your own sexuality and overcoming sexual problems is to understand what ideas you have learnt about sexual feelings and behaviour, and where these ideas have come from. We learn about sex directly from what other people say to us or from what we read and see. We also learn about sex indirectly through the 'messages' we receive in what people say or don't say, or in what they do or don't do. For example, a child who has her hand slapped when she is touching her genitals might feel she is

doing something wrong and shameful. This is one of the messages she has received about sexual behaviour.

The exercise below helps you to find out what messages you received about sex and to discover the thoughts and feelings about sex and your own sexuality that you learnt as you grew up. Before doing this exercise, read through all the instructions and the example.

Exercise: Messages about sex

Relax and let your mind reflect back over your childhood and teenage years. Think about the messages you received about sex. Write down the name of the first person who comes to mind who gave you a message about sex. Then write down what that message was. Next write down the name of another person and the message they gave you. Continue doing this until you cannot think of any more. You might name an individual person or a group of people. You may have learnt messages about sex from the internet or social media, from sexting that went wrong, revenge porn or being shamed for your body or sexual activity on social media. You will have received some message about sex from your abuser. Put this message on your list if you can. If you find it too distressing to think about, leave the abuser out of this exercise for the moment.

Example: Polly's messages about sex

Person	Message
Mother	'Never spoke about sex, changed the TV channel when bed scenes came on. The message I got was sex is shameful and embarrassing.'
Teacher	'In sex education lessons, we learnt about rabbits, sperm, eggs and conception. The message I got was that sex was a cold and clinical subject to do with biology, not feelings.'
Ex-boyfriend	'Shared photos of me naked on social media after we split up. Sent them to all our friends. The message I got was "You are a dirty slut" for exposing your body.'
Abuser	'Raped me. The message I got was that sex is something that's done to me. I have no control or right to refuse it. How I feel sexually doesn't matter.'

Boyfriend   'Said I was cold and not very romantic. I got the
               message that I was sexually inadequate, that there
               was something wrong with me.'

Exercise: Challenging the myths and negative messages

Look at your list of messages about sex. Try to challenge any
negative messages or thoughts about sex by writing the negative
thoughts down on one side of a piece of paper, and more reasonable or positive responses to these thoughts down the other.

Example

Negative thoughts	Reasonable thoughts
'I have no control over sex or right to refuse it.'	'It's my body. I have a right to say "No" to sex.'
'Sex is embarrassing and shameful.'	'Sex is natural. Some people are embarrassed about it, but it doesn't have to be that way. I can learn to feel more relaxed about the subject.'
'I am a dirty slut.'	'Being intimate with the person you care about is normal.'
'Sex is dirty.'	'What's dirty about it? It's natural.'

Notice which negative messages are influencing your feelings,
thoughts and behaviour now. Learning to challenge these negative
thoughts and replace them with more realistic thinking, is the first
step towards a more positive attitude.

LEARNING ABOUT YOUR BODY AND SEX

Having knowledge about how your body works and about sexual
activity is important in overcoming sexual difficulties. Fear thrives
on ignorance. Fight your fear with knowledge and by learning to
love and accept your body.

- Do the body image exercises recommended in Chapter 10. Learn
  to accept all your body, including the bits you may have avoided
  looking at, especially the sexual parts.
- Find some books or leaflets to read with good clear information
  about your body and sexuality. Challenge the myths you have
  learnt with some facts. Challenge the negative messages with

positive information. Look at the book lists on DABS' website (at: <www.dabs.uk.com>).

- Search for information on sex education on the internet, but be careful you do not click on any pornography sites.

The survivors' group has also changed me. Now I cannot learn enough about the way it feels in body and mind when making love with someone special and so I have read a few books on sex. To say they were an eye-opener is an understatement. The effect they had on me was enormous. I always thought there was me, the one who doesn't really know how to behave or what to feel and there is man – the mystery, the enigma. The first book I read, *Making Love*, turned out to be a book for men with sexual problems. In my ignorance I thought a man was always ready, willing and able to have sex and orgasm after orgasm. As I read, I understood that men are not all that different from women. They worry about the size of their penis as we do about the size or shape of our breasts. I had put men and sex on a pedestal to look up to and be in awe of. Now I understand that they have the same fears, worries and insecurities about their bodies and performance during sex. How could I ever hope to enjoy the relaxation needed for good sex if I pull in my stomach to make it look flatter? Or worry whether he has noticed a stretchmark or would he notice my thighs are too fat when he gives me oral sex? How many men worried about whether they were good enough for me when we had sex while I was nervous about whether I was touching and moving in the right way? The books I read made me feel an equal to the man. I realize how important communication is in lovemaking and how essential it is to feel relaxed in body and mind.
Katarina

LEARNING TO COMMUNICATE
Learning to communicate more openly about sex and your feelings is essential in resolving sexual difficulties. Many people do not know what words to use for the sexual parts of men's and women's bodies and for sexual activities, and this makes it hard to talk about sex. Some words may seem too crude and others too clinical.

Exercise: Language of sex
Write down all the words you can think of to describe the female genitals (for example, vagina, pussy, cunt), the male genitals (for

example, penis, cock) and sexual intercourse (for example, fuck, make love, screw).

Choose the words you want to use and say the words out loud until you feel comfortable with them. If you have a partner, practise saying the words out loud with your partner until it becomes easy. It's hard to talk about sex if you don't have any words to use.

FOLLOW YOUR FEELINGS

You have a right to say 'Yes' or 'No' to being touched by another person or to having sex with them. It is your body and your choice. As a child, you may have been unable to say 'No' to being touched, or to having sex, and you may still feel that you do not have a choice. Many survivors think that they *must* touch or have sex with another person even when they don't want to because:

- the other person wants to;
- the other person is sexually excited;
- it's their duty;
- they've already responded to the kisses and cuddles;
- other people's feelings are more important than their own;
- the other person has been nice to them;
- the other person will be bad-tempered/upset/aggressive if they don't.

These thoughts may have been learnt from being abused. Jane learnt to give in to sex to avoid her stepfather's anger. You don't have to have sex, touch someone else or be touched unless *you* want to and choose to. This is your right whatever the circumstances. However, you may not feel able to exercise this right if you are afraid of the consequences, feel guilty or are being threatened or overpowered.

Many survivors feel anxious about sex because they begin to feel powerless, out of control and physically invaded again. Ultimately, it can only be damaging to your own sexual feelings or relationship to have sex with someone when you don't want to. Learning to make a choice about what you do, and what you don't do, based on *your own* feelings is a way of treating yourself and the other person with respect. It also helps you feel more in control of your own body and your own life.

While you are trying to deal with your feelings about being

sexually abused, you may find you do not want to have sex or any physical contact at all. Follow what you are feeling. Listen to your body. If you feel uncomfortable with someone, you probably do not want any physical or sexual contact. This is your right. If you have a partner, explain how you are feeling and ask him or her to respect your wishes. These feelings do not have to last for ever. Reassure your partner that this is part of the healing process. Many sexual problems arise because people do not speak about what they are really feeling, or act on those feelings; instead they pretend to their partner, or do what they think their partner wants them to do.

LEARNING TO RELAX

Learning to relax is essential for dealing with sexual difficulties. Tension prevents the experience of sexual feelings and pleasure. You may have learnt from the abuse to tense your body automatically when you are in any sexual situation and when you begin to have sexual feelings.

Learn to relax in non-sexual situations to begin with. Learn to notice the difference between feeling relaxed and feeling tense. Notice where you hold tension in your body and what causes that tension to begin or to get worse. Next, start to apply these techniques to sexual situations. Try to relax; notice whereabouts in your body you are holding any tension and what caused the tension to start. Many survivors discover that they automatically tense their bodies as soon as their partner hugs or kisses them, or as soon as they begin to feel aroused.

TOUCHING YOURSELF

Survivors often feel uncomfortable about their own bodies and try to avoid thinking about them, looking at them or touching them. They may have negative feelings about their bodies because their bodies were the focus of the abuse. Learning to enjoy touching yourself is a way of exploring and overcoming these negative feelings and learning to love and accept your own body. Read through the exercise below before attempting it. Be aware that it might bring up negative feelings, and recognize and accept these feelings. Discovering what sorts of touches bring up bad feelings can be helpful.

Exercise

This exercise does not have to be done in one sitting. Do it a little at a time and stop when you want to or if you feel too distressed. Come back to the exercise when you feel ready. Make some time when you can be on your own and feel relaxed. Find somewhere comfortable to lie or sit and then slowly begin to explore your own body by touching and stroking it or maybe gently massaging it with oil. Start with a part of your body that feels safe, maybe your face, feet or hands. Try different types of touching; gentle, firm, tickling, slow or fast. Notice your feelings as you are doing this and what feels good and what doesn't feel good. Move to another 'safe' part of your body and repeat this process. Gradually, work through all the parts of your body in this way. Leave your breasts and genitals, or any areas that you feel anxious about, until last. Only attempt these areas when you feel ready and when you can relax and feel comfortable and safe.

As you are doing this exercise, be aware of what gives you pleasure. Notice if you begin to feel tense or anxious with any type of touching or any part of your body. Does this remind you of anything that happened when you were abused? Notice any disturbing thoughts, images, feelings or memories that come up and write them down as soon as you can. This exercise can help you learn about your own body and feelings and so begin to understand and appreciate your own sexuality. This is a basic foundation for learning to feel comfortable with masturbation or a sexual relationship with another person.

GIVING AND RECEIVING TOUCHES

When you have completed the exercise on touching yourself, you can then go on to repeat a similar exercise with your partner (if you have one). The exercise is aimed at helping you feel safe and comfortable with touching your partner and being touched. It also helps partners to communicate about what feels good or bad.

Exercise

The exercise below is in two parts and may take a number of sessions over a few weeks or months to complete. You must go at your own pace and not try to rush through the exercise.

Before beginning this exercise, make a pact with your partner that you will not have sexual intercourse or genital contact during the exercise sessions. You may feel safer and more relaxed when you know that touching will not lead to full sex.

Find a time when you and your partner won't be disturbed, and choose a warm and comfortable place to do this exercise. Find a way to relax together, perhaps by doing a relaxation exercise or listening to music, but avoid using alcohol or drugs. Ask your partner to touch the part of your body that feels the most comfortable and safe to you (for example, your hands, arms or feet). Relax and simply accept the touches. Ask your partner to vary the speed and firmness of the touches and tell him or her what feels good and what doesn't. Repeat this exercise for different parts of your body. Take your time, and gradually work towards the parts of your body that you have felt less comfortable about being touched. Only ask your partner to touch these parts of your body when you feel safe and ready for this.

Reverse the roles and become the person who gives the touches while your partner relaxes. Start with the part of your partner's body that you feel most safe and comfortable with. Tell your partner how you are feeling as you are touching him or her. Repeat this exercise for different parts of your partner's body, gradually working towards the parts you feel most uneasy about. This part of the exercise is for *you* to look at your thoughts and feelings about touching someone else. Some survivors have more difficulty in touching their partner than in being touched themselves. However, you might also want to ask your partner to tell you how he or she feels about the different types of touching you are giving.

Throughout these exercises, notice how you are feeling. If you begin to feel anxious, tense or uncomfortable, stop or ask your partner to stop. Relax and let any feelings, thoughts or memories come to the surface. Write them down and discuss as much as you want to with your partner. Go back to that area of the body or that type of touch only when you feel more comfortable about it.

This exercise enables survivors to gradually work through any negative feelings about being touched or touching in a safe and relaxed atmosphere. It also helps partners to start to communicate about what feels pleasurable and what doesn't. Often partners have never done this and may have guessed incorrectly what the other person likes or dislikes. Learning to communicate openly in this way can help to break down anger, resentment and hurt that may have built up in the relationship.

If it is difficult for you to say 'Stop', or to say that you don't like something, agree a code word or gesture beforehand and use that instead.

DEALING WITH FLASHBACKS

Flashbacks can be very distressing and frightening for survivors, and confusing to a partner, when they happen during sex. If your partner does not already know what happens when you have a flashback, explain it to him or her as soon as you can. When a flashback happens, stop whatever you are doing and tell your partner that you are having a flashback. Then ask your partner to help you follow the four steps below. You can also follow these steps when you have a flashback and are on your own.

- Grounding – remind yourself how old you are, where you are and who you are with. Look around the room and name the objects in the room. Keep reminding yourself that you aren't a child with the abuser but an adult who is safe now (for example, I am 27; I have my own home in Westfield Close; I am with my husband Mike; I can see my wardrobe, my hairbrush, my shoes; the abuser is *not* here; I am safe).
- Find out what triggered the flashback – a word, a phrase, a smell, a touch, a certain type of sex or a certain sexual position. Tell your partner.
- If you were having sex and want to continue, do so. If you feel bad, and don't want to, don't.
- Make a note of the memory you had in the flashbacks as soon as you are able to do so. Flashbacks have the power to frighten you when you try to push the memories away. Keep writing down your flashbacks, drawing them or expressing the content in other ways as this can also help.
- Flashbacks occur when unprocessed material from a traumatic incident of sexual abuse is triggered and it feels as if the incident is replaying again now. EMDR or other trauma-focused therapies can help you process and resolve the traumatic material fairly quickly (see 'Sources of help' at the back of the book to find a therapist).

Summary

Many survivors of child abuse experience sexual difficulties as teenagers and adults. This is a result of the process of 'traumatic sexualization' that the survivor has experienced as a child. The resulting sexual difficulties and responses range from a preoccupation with sex and sexual matters, to fear and avoidance of sex and relationships.

Some survivors feel confused or fearful about their sexual orientation. Survivors often find that their sexual difficulties and responses vary at different times of their life. Flashbacks, seeing the abuser's face superimposed on your partner's face, and other disturbing body sensations and emotional reactions, are a direct result of the sexual trauma experienced during the sexual abuse getting 'stuck' in the brain and being triggered in the present.

Overcoming sexual difficulties begins with working on feelings of guilt and shame about the sexual abuse. It also involves allowing yourself time to understand, explore and develop your sexual knowledge and experience, in a way that was denied to you as a child. Difficulties with sex and sexuality are part of a bigger problem and cannot be tackled in isolation.

Dealing with sexual difficulties involves looking at emotional and physical health, relationship problems, myths and negative attitudes to sex, knowledge and understanding about bodies and sexual matters, and ways of communicating about sex. You can learn to understand and feel more positive about your body and about physical and sexual closeness. You can learn to feel in control, to relax and to enjoy sexual experiences on your own or with a partner.

Suggestions

- To explore your sexual feelings and overcome any difficulties, follow the suggestions and do the exercises described in this chapter.
- Try reading a book from the 'Recovery' section of the book list on DABS' website (at: <www.dabs.uk.com>).
- Relate (at: <www.relate.org.uk>) can help with relationship and sexual problems, whether or not you have a partner.

Part 4
FEELINGS TOWARDS OTHERS

12

Children

Survivors sometimes find that they have difficulties in relating to children, both their own children and children in general. They may find they have no feelings for their children, cannot touch them, or feel angry and hostile towards them. Other survivors feel anxious and fearful for children and overprotect them, or feel out of control and unable to cope. This chapter discusses the links between being sexually abused as a child and having problems with children as an adult, and then looks at some of the problems in more detail and suggests ways of overcoming them.

Fiona's story

As I carried my baby I was frightened I would not be able to love it. When Amy was born, I overprotected her. I wouldn't let her out of my sight nor let anyone do anything for her. She was mine, the first human I could love. I had a terrible fear of losing her and this made me depressed. I worried about her all the time and I was afraid to leave her with people in case she was abused.

I decided she wasn't going to be like me. She had to be perfectly clean and tidy and so the house she lived in had to be too. This became an obsession with me. Even her hair had to be perfect. I'd blow it dry every morning. I'd buy clothes for her and then wouldn't let her wear them in case they got dirty. I washed her if she got the least bit dirty. I cared too much about what other people thought about me and Amy. I chastised her when I thought other people would think that was the right thing to do. I got to the stage where I didn't know what was wrong and what was right. If I smacked her in front of others for doing something naughty then afterwards I felt that they thought I was a bad mother. If I didn't smack her I felt that they would talk about her and wouldn't like her.

I wanted so much for everyone to like her but often I convinced myself they didn't, so I would push her away. My moods were always changing. I used to explode at her then feel that I was wicked and a bad parent. I would get so depressed. Even though I have never physically abused her, I was always afraid: 'What if I explode next time and hurt her?' So I would avoid chastising her and she would only have to cry and she got her own way. I tried so hard to be a perfect mother but the pressure would get too much and I would erupt again and then sink into a depression.

I'd have wrapped her up in cotton wool if I could. If other children teased her, it would really hurt. I'd imagine Amy to be feeling like I felt as a child, 'No one likes me'. I used to get so mixed up, and confused my own emotions with Amy's. It was hard to cuddle my child because I never knew what was wrong or right. I'd feel guilty and afraid people might think I was abusing her. Because of all these obsessions my daughter became very clingy towards me. Again I imagined she felt like I did as a child so I wouldn't want to leave her. I believed she couldn't bear to be without me. I'd get irritable and angry when she'd cry after me.

I dreaded her starting school even when she was a baby. What would I do without her? I'd get so depressed and worry about her. I was always living in the future. I avoided playing with her and was afraid to enjoy her company because I knew she would go to school one day. I was tormented with the thought that she was lonely the way I had been. I thought of having another child as company for her but I knew I couldn't cope with another one. I felt really guilty and so sorry for her that I spoilt her to make up for it.

As time goes on I am beginning to get better and my obsessions are slowly going. I no longer chastise her for other people's sake but for what I think is right or wrong. I cuddle my daughter without fear. I know I would never hurt her. Now she is 7 and I can explain my outbursts to her, telling her that it isn't her fault. I am working on all the other problems, which are smaller now. She has been affected by all this but with time and care I know I can put it right. We have a very special relationship. She isn't clingy. I know she can survive without me being there to protect her all the time. I enjoy the freedom when she is at school and she enjoys school. I am learning to be assertive with her and to realize she is not me. She never will suffer abuse and pain the way I did. She is a happy little girl.

Fiona's story illustrates many of the difficulties that survivors experience with children.

Sexual abuse and problems with children:
making the links

Below we discuss three consequences of being sexually abused that can lead to problems with children: being reminded of the abuse, feeling very needy, and the lack of a good model of parenting. Making the links between their present problems with children and their own past sexual abuse is the first step for survivors in trying to understand and change their relationships with children.

BEING REMINDED OF THE ABUSE

> Something very surprising happened to me a few days ago. I went to buy my daughter some shoes and while she looked through the shelves, I sat on a low seat. A man came in with a little girl holding his hand. She was about 2 years old. They stood next to me and I was at eye-level with the child. We looked at each other, holding each other's eyes. Her eyes looked old, knowing. I wondered if she was being abused, and thought, 'maybe not now, maybe in 2 years'. I was 4 when I was abused. I saw myself in the child. I looked at her eyes and cried. I did not sob, but my tears flowed relentlessly. **Katarina**

Survivors often try to bury their painful memories and feelings about their abuse. When survivors are with children, this way of coping can break down because the children remind them of their own childhood and the sexual abuse. This can cause survivors to have difficulties spending time with children. Forgotten memories and feelings about sexual abuse are triggered, particularly by children who in some way remind the survivor of him- or herself as a child: children of the same age the survivor was when the abuse started; children who look and act like the survivor as a child; or children who have been sexually abused. Survivors with babies are often reminded of their own vulnerability when a child, and of their own abuse. Survivors may be disturbed and reminded of their own abuse by seeing a baby boy's erection, a young girl playing with her genitals, or signs of an older child's developing sexuality.

Ingrid was reminded of her abuse and experienced intense feelings of fear when her son reached the age her abuser was when the abuse started.

Although I could feel love for my daughters, I felt mainly indifference towards my son. But when he grew into a teenager, the age my abuser was when he abused me and threatened me, I began to fear him. **Ingrid**

SURVIVORS' NEEDINESS

Survivors were often very needy as children because they were not protected or understood and did not have their feelings looked after. Adult survivors who are still very needy themselves are often unable to meet their children's needs, or attempt to compensate for their own neediness by trying to give their children everything they did not have themselves. Both these reactions can cause problems in relating to children.

Survivors often find that they do not have the emotional or physical energy to meet their children's demands and to give the care and attention that is needed. A child's demands can feel overwhelming for survivors who are having to cope with their own emotions and difficulties. They may emotionally withdraw from their children or be unable to provide a happy and stimulating atmosphere. Some survivors find even the physical demands of feeding, dressing and washing a child are more than they can cope with.

Problems are also caused by survivors trying to compensate for their own neediness through their children. Fiona had never been clean as a child so she tried to keep Amy absolutely clean all the time. Fiona had often felt lonely as a child so she spoilt Amy when she thought Amy felt lonely. But Fiona's 'compensation' did not help Amy because Fiona was not responding to Amy's feelings or needs but to her own childhood feelings. She was trying, through Amy, to put right the things that had been wrong for her when she was a child.

LACK OF A GOOD PARENTING MODEL

People usually learn the basic ideas of parenting from their own parents' behaviour. Survivors who have been sexually abused by parents, and sometimes physically and emotionally abused as well, may find they have difficulty in parenting because they have never learnt basic skills that others take for granted.

Survivors may feel so anxious about how to be a good parent that they feel paralysed by uncertainty or try to copy others. Survivors may sometimes repeat their parents' poor behaviour (for example, by not listening to a child or threatening the child with being taken into care) without realizing the effect they are having on the child. More commonly, survivors are so desperate not to repeat the abusive parenting they themselves suffered that they go to the opposite extreme – allowing children to do anything they want to, avoiding physical contact with them and never saying 'No' to the children.

Problems in relation to children

Box 9 lists some of the problems survivors experience with children. Following it, we discuss some of the main ones in more detail.

Box 9 Difficulties in relation to children

- Excessive fear for children's safety.
- Overprotecting children.
- Inappropriately protecting children.
- Rejecting children.
- Anger and hostility towards children.
- Not being able to show love and affection to children.
- Not being able to touch children.
- Over-controlling children.
- Having difficulties with children of a particular age.
- Physically abusing children.
- Emotionally abusing children.
- Verbally abusing children.
- Sexually abusing children.
- Overindulging children.
- Not being able to assert your own needs with children.
- Not being able to say 'No' to children.
- Feeling helpless and out of control with children.
- Not feeling love for your own children.
- Not being able to bath children.
- Excessively washing children.
- Being unable to cope with a child being upset/hurt/angry.
- Confusing own feelings with the child's.

NO FEELINGS

Some survivors find that they do not feel love for their children or are unable to give the emotional care and support a child needs. Below, Ingrid describes her lack of feeling for her son.

My son was born and when I saw him for the first time, I felt nothing. No joy, but no resentment either. 'Well,' I thought, 'maybe mother-love comes later.' I tried to be the kind of mother I had seen in others, but the mother-love never came. I did like him most of the time but equally felt no need to have him close to me. I had no understanding of the needs of a child. I fed him, clothed him and gave him material things, but I did not nurture him emotionally. I had nothing to guide me and no emotions to give. I never hit him but I never showed him love either. I was glad when my son stopped coming to me, looking for love and affection.

Sometimes I felt sorry for him and tried to pull myself together and play with him or read him a story. But within minutes I felt as if something inside me was screaming to get away from him. I felt imprisoned and crowded. I knew that I had to share myself with him, give him part of myself, but there was so little left. So much had been taken away from me by abuse, humiliation and hurt. There was a small part of me in which I had made my little haven of peace by blocking out emotions and feelings. I felt this little part would now be invaded by this child and I would be forced to acknowledge feelings of some kind. **Ingrid**

Ingrid was unable to love her son because she had tried to forget about her abuse and had pushed away her feelings. In burying her bad feelings, she had also buried her ability to love and feel happy and close to someone. Ingrid felt threatened by her son and felt that if she opened herself up and started loving him, she might also open up her feelings about her abuse. She was very needy and felt she had so little left of herself that her son might take it all away.

Ingrid had not been given the emotional care she had needed as a child and did not have the parenting skills to cope with her son. Like Ingrid, survivors may be unable to feel anything for their children, or may simply not know how to give emotional care and love if they have never experienced this themselves. The child who does not receive the love he or she needs may become overanxious and clingy, angry and badly behaved or cut off and emotionally withdrawn.

AVOIDING TOUCH

> I still remember the relief I felt when my six-year-old son asked me not to hold his hand in the street any more, because he was a 'big boy' now. From that day onwards, I used that excuse not to touch him physically. I think the last time I kissed him was when he was about five or six years old. **Ingrid**

Some survivors avoid physical contact with their children. They may avoid hugging, kissing or holding hands with the child, and refuse to bathe the child or have the child sit on their knee. When survivors are very needy themselves, or are emotionally distressed, a child wanting to be hugged and kissed can feel like another demand that they are unable to meet. Survivors who are withdrawn or depressed may find it hard to express physical affection, and survivors who have no feelings for their children or feel hostile towards them may not want to.

Physical contact between a survivor, as an adult, and a child may bring back memories and feelings about the abuse. In pushing the child away, the survivor is pushing away those memories and feelings. Survivors who sometimes physically reject children may at other times be able to show love and affection, and overcompensate at these times by pulling the child towards them and hugging and loving them profusely. This see-saw between physical rejection and compensating 'over-loving' can be very confusing and hurtful to a child.

Survivors may also be unsure about what kind of touching is right for a parent or adult to give a child. Is it normal to hug, kiss or stroke a child; or is it abuse? Is it normal to bathe a child, or be in bed with a child, or hold a child when the parent is naked; or is it abuse? Survivors who have been abused by their own parents are more likely to have these worries and may feel so frightened of abusing that they stop touching their children altogether.

> It is natural to play with your baby but it felt wrong to me, like I was interfering with her. I couldn't cuddle her without feeling bad about it. I loved Lynn very much and she needed to know that, but I just couldn't show her. So Lynn was isolated in her own little world. She was also always putting her arms around strangers. Now I find Lynn either won't leave me alone or doesn't come near me at all. **Sally**

As a child, Graham had no father and was sexually abused and betrayed in many ways by his mother. He never learnt what a parent–child relationship should be like, but he did learn that physical contact with his mother always resulted in sexual abuse. This has affected his relationship with his own children:

> I find it difficult to talk to my children or play with them and I can't cuddle them or show love and affection. **Graham**

An unfortunate consequence of the growth in awareness of child sexual abuse is that many fathers, whether survivors or not, avoid bathing and cuddling their children because they are scared of being seen as abusers. Survivors are particularly afraid that they will be seen as abusers so may avoid all physical contact with children. The myth that all survivors become abusers makes some survivors fear they will suddenly start abusing their children. The majority of survivors, however, have a strong desire to protect children and would never touch a child sexually. Children can be distressed by parents avoiding touching, cuddling and kissing them. They may feel anxious or angry, or become clingy or withdrawn.

ANGER AND REJECTION

> There I was, finally I had a baby. All mine, all I'd ever wanted, a baby. 'Congratulations, it's a boy!' Why was I crying? I'd got my wish come true but I wanted a girl.
>
> I was just so happy at first to have a baby that I soon got over it being a boy. Two years later I was in the middle of a nervous breakdown. I hated my two-year-old son. I couldn't stand the sight of him. I hated men of all descriptions. I felt that they were full of demands, especially my son as he couldn't do anything himself. 'I want my breakfast now, Mum, please,' is a pretty normal request in anybody's eyes, but the 'I want' syndrome grated on my brain. Everybody always seemed to be wanting, but nobody said 'What do you want? How do you feel? What do you want to do?' or even, 'Thank you.'
>
> As I became more depressed I couldn't bring myself to do anything but the necessaries like give my son breakfast, dinner, tea and so on. I couldn't love him, cuddle him, play with him, be interested in any way in him or spend time with him. I didn't even want to be in the same room with him for any length of

time. This lasted until my husband pointed out that I was being a rotten mother to my son and he would grow up hating me.

One day my son had done something wrong (hardly surprising since he spent all day, every day, playing alone in his bedroom, out of my sight) and I went to town on him and couldn't stop smacking him. If my husband hadn't come home when he did I would have probably smacked my son so much that it would have been classed as physical abuse. I sat on the landing in my husband's arms shouting and screaming, 'I swore I'd never beat my kids like my father beat me.'

My husband then made me realize I needed help. I went to a group for adults who were sexually abused as children. Talking to other women and mothers, I found out I wasn't the only one who felt this way or treated their children this way. I realized the reason I hated my son so much was the fact that he was a boy, and I was frightened of him becoming an abuser. I'd just never understood this before. **Pam**

Pam was trying to meet the demands of a 2-year-old child when she had not sorted out her feelings about her sexual abuse, and was in great need of care and support herself. As with Ingrid, Pam's own neediness interfered with her ability to meet her child's needs and she felt angry and resentful about his demands. Pam saw her son as a potential abuser and was angry at him for reminding her of the past abuse.

Underneath her depression, Pam hid a huge well of anger about her own childhood, her abuse and the abuser. These buried feelings of anger were beginning to surface, and Pam was directing them at her son. Children are always easy targets for anger and hostility. They are smaller and less powerful than an adult and usually forgive their parents' outbursts. Survivors may vent feelings on children that they are too frightened to express elsewhere – anger is expressed at a small son but not at the abuser. Some survivors are angry and hostile towards their children because they do not know any other way of being in control. This may have been the only form of discipline they saw from their own parents. Many survivors want to love and care for their children but do not know how to overcome their bad feelings or change their behaviour.

Anger and rejection towards a child can lead to problems in the child such as bedwetting, temper tantrums, running away or sullen or clingy behaviour. The survivor may find herself unable to cope with these problems and feel even more anger and resentment towards the child.

OVERPROTECTING

I'm always worried about my children and I overprotect them. **Graham**

Many survivors find themselves overprotecting their children because they are frightened that they will be sexually abused as well. This may involve keeping the child in the house, not allowing him or her to do normal childhood things, shouting at the child for showing physical affection, making sure the child keeps his or her body well covered at all times, and not allowing the child to play with other children or go on school trips. A survivor may not react in the same way with all of his or her children. Some survivors overprotect girls but not boys. Survivors are particularly likely to overprotect any child who reminds them of themselves as children.

Sally's eldest daughter Lynn looks and acts very much like Sally did as a child. Sally feels Lynn is a vulnerable child who is destined to be abused.

I was very protective with Lynn and still am at times. No one is allowed to come near her, I am always so afraid that she is in danger from others. **Sally**

She acts much more strictly with Lynn than with her younger daughter and gets extremely angry if Lynn hugs or kisses Sally's male friends.

Ingrid had been abused by her brother and because of this tried to protect her daughters from males in the family.

I have to be very careful not to destroy my family life. The suspicion I hold against my son and my husband, whenever they get close to my daughters, is tearing me apart. If my son suggests a game of chess in his room with his sister, I have to force myself not to interfere because I see the abuser getting me into the bedroom under a pretence. Because of the abuse, I have destroyed any beginnings of a normal brother–sister relationship because I tried to separate them whenever possible. For the first years I did not realize what I was doing. When I did realize, I forced myself to stop, not always with success. If one of my daughters sits on my husband's lap, I have to keep my eyes away because I cannot bear to watch what it might lead to (or would have led to had it been me and my abuser). Often I have to go out of the room.

While I was watching and worrying about my own family, my youngest daughter was sexually abused by a neighbour. She did not tell me until three years after the abuse. **Ingrid**

Ingrid was being reminded of her own abuse. She was responding to her own feelings of vulnerability and fear about being abused rather than usefully and realistically protecting her children. She did not concern herself with the danger from people outside the family because this had not been her experience. This kind of protection – seeing danger for specific children only or from a specific type of person – is inappropriate and does not guarantee children's safety.

Louise was enraged when her daughter Rebecca showed her knickers while doing a somersault at a children's party. Rebecca was smacked and sent home. Louise still blamed herself for being abused as a child and felt she had provoked the abuse by not keeping her body properly covered up. She was frightened by Rebecca's behaviour, and smacked her because she did not want her to be abused and did not know how else to protect her.

I know children have always done somersaults and that my reaction to Rebecca showing her pants was extreme. I try to hide it, but I live in constant fear of her exposing herself and perhaps creating the conditions that caused me to be abused as a child. **Louise**

Louise's attempt to protect Rebecca was inappropriate. Rebecca was not putting herself in danger by showing her knickers; people don't suddenly abuse because they see a child's knickers.

Children and young people are vulnerable and need to be protected in appropriate ways. Survivors, however, often overprotect their children and young people in ways that are restrictive and stifling, and that can cause difficulties for the child. Inappropriate protection may leave children and young people feeling confused or ashamed, and does not help to keep them safe from abuse.

NO CONTROL
Elspeth did not like to say 'No' to her children and spoil their fun. She let them do whatever they wanted to do. They were always

climbing on her, pulling at her, demanding her attention and asking for sweets and presents. Elspeth became worn out, and her children became more and more unruly. Every so often, Elspeth's patience snapped and she shouted and screamed at her children and then felt terribly guilty. She would cry and tell her children she was sorry over and over again and buy them sweets to make up. Elspeth felt helpless and out of control.

Elspeth had been physically and sexually abused as a child by her father. She had grown up feeling frightened and lacking in self-confidence, and did not want her own children to grow up like this. She was so frightened of treating her own children badly that she did not put any restrictions on them at all. Elspeth was trying to make up for the abuse she had suffered as a child through her own children. She had never experienced parents treating children firmly but fairly, and she did not know how to be assertive.

Like Elspeth, many survivors are so anxious to make their children's childhoods different from their own that they allow their own feelings and needs to be trampled on. As children and young people, survivors were deprived of their rights when they were being abused. As adults, survivors may not know how to assert themselves or may feel they have no right to do so.

> I was totally unable to assert myself with my children. It was very difficult for me to ask them to help with any housework. Sometimes I forced myself to ask meekly if one of them would be kind enough to wash the dishes or vacuum the carpet. It was very, very difficult for me and I could only do it after apologizing profusely. If they refused, I gave up and ended up doing it myself, biting back the tears of humiliation about being treated like a maid. **Katarina**

Survivors often find it hard to trust other people and lack friendships and close relationships. They sometimes feel that the only people they can trust and love completely are their own children, and are very anxious not to jeopardize these relationships. They may be fearful of making any demands on their children, saying 'No' to them or putting any limits on what they can do, in case they lose their children's love.

Like Elspeth and Katarina, many survivors feel out of control with their children or worn down by continually trying to meet their demands. Problems will develop between survivors and their children if survivors do not teach their children the difference between acceptable and unacceptable behaviour.

DEPRIVED OF CHILDREN

Sexual abuse can result in some women being unable to have children because they have been physically damaged by sexually transmitted diseases, forced sexual intercourse, sexual torture or insertion of objects into their vaginas. This can leave them infertile, prone to miscarriages or in need of a hysterectomy. Sexual abuse also causes emotional damage that may make survivors decide not to have children because they think they will not be able to cope, or because they fear 'passing on' their problems to their own children. At one time, Rhys thought he would not be able to have children because he was concerned about the effect his own childhood abuse would have on his relationships with children.

> I never wanted children. Now I have a son and I love him so much. I live for him. **Rhys**

Rhys overcame his fears and has a very good relationship with his son.

Luke did want children but had to work on concerns arising from his own abuse before he could become a father.

> I always wanted children but I had anxieties and worries about having children. I was able to discuss my worries openly and freely with my partner. I now have children and I love it. **Luke**

Some survivors are deprived of having children because of their fears of relationships or sexual intercourse. Being deprived of children in these ways can be a further cause of grief and anger for survivors, and can cause feelings of resentment and jealousy towards parents and their children.

Some survivors who do have children are unable to cope with looking after them because of the emotional problems they have themselves or because of difficulties with the child. They may have to allow other people to take over care of the child temporarily or permanently, or have the child taken into care. Survivors may miss out on stages of their children's lives, and feel guilty for not being able to cope or not being a good enough parent. Having children taken into care or losing custody of children can feel like a further punishment or abuse.

SEXUALLY ABUSED CHILDREN

Ingrid had been sexually abused as a child and recently discovered that her daughter, Rosie aged 8, had also been abused a few years previously.

> When my youngest daughter told me she had been sexually abused, I developed eczema on both my legs within hours. I started scratching it until it bled and in the days that followed opened the wounds again and again. I did not know if I could cope. Would I be strong enough, not only for myself but also for her? I felt ashamed of myself and my lack of self-control. I realized what I was doing but I could not stop. Scratching my eczema had been my only way of coping with my suffering as a child. I was coping in the same way again. **Ingrid**

Rosie's abuse brought back disturbing memories and feelings for Ingrid but, because Ingrid had attended a survivors' group, she could cope and was able to support Rosie without blaming her.

Fiona also discovered that her daughter Amy had been sexually abused by two neighbourhood boys.

> The day I found out what had been happening must have been the worst day of my life. At the time, I was still in therapy myself and I was very sensitive to it all. I kept calm although I wanted to scream at her. I was loving and supporting, although at that time I disliked her and my overwhelming instinct and desire was to run away, to get away from her. The whole situation had brought up things I didn't want to cope with. I saw my daughter the way I saw myself all those years ago. She was dirty, ruined and no good. She was like a damaged toy. I couldn't handle this. I'd protected her and worked hard all those years to make sure my daughter wouldn't be like me. **Fiona**

Fiona felt the same disgust for Amy that she had felt for herself, but she was at least able to outwardly support and accept Amy. In therapy, Fiona worked through her own feelings about herself, and she stopped blaming Amy when she stopped blaming herself for the abuse.

> Now, 18 months on, Amy and I talk openly about it all. I now trust her and know she would tell me if anything ever happened

again. I am learning that what happened to me many years ago wasn't my fault, just like it wasn't Amy's fault. It seemed like the end of the world when Amy told me. I never believed I could love her or that things would be normal between us again. Now I have dealt with my worst fear and the whole situation has helped bring up things about myself and by dealing with them I am a stronger person. **Fiona**

Survivors who discover their own child has been abused have to deal with their feelings about both their child's abuse and the memories and feelings about their own abuse. Survivors who are teachers, health visitors or social workers, or work with children and young people in any way, are also likely to come in contact with sexually abused children, and may have difficulties in dealing with this. The survivor may feel angry and hostile towards sexually abused children for reminding him or her of their own abuse, or for disclosing the abuse when the survivor had kept silent. The survivor may cope by ignoring the child's abuse, or feel powerless to protect the child and consequently do nothing. Survivors who still blame themselves for being abused may also blame abused children and young people they meet. Dealing with a sexually abused child can be traumatic for survivors who have not worked through the issues resulting from their own abuse. A survivor who has helped and healed him- or herself is in a position to help and support an abused child with strength and confidence.

Overcoming the problems

Working through this book, getting therapy and talking to other people about your sexual abuse will generally help you feel better and improve your relationships with children and young people. Below we discuss ways in which you can work on overcoming your problems with children by remembering the abuse, dealing with your own neediness and learning to be a more confident parent.

REMEMBERING THE ABUSE
Trying to forget the abuse is a coping strategy that does not work for long and makes you vulnerable to being suddenly reminded of your abuse and childhood emotions. Children may remind you of your own abuse, and this can cause problems unless you are willing

to face your memories and feelings by allowing them to surface and dealing with them.

Exercise

When you are with children and young people, try to observe your own thoughts and feelings. Notice whether they remind you of yourself or of your earlier abuse. Take note of any strong feelings (anger, distress, fear) that you have when you are with children. As soon as you can, write down your observations and any childhood memories and feelings that have surfaced.

Observing your own feelings, memories and behaviour, and writing them down, will help you sort out which feelings relate to your own childhood abuse and which are about the children you are with. Getting therapy for yourself or talking to other survivors can also help this process.

SURVIVORS' NEEDINESS

Many survivors hate who they were as children. Try to understand and accept the child that you were at the time when you were being sexually abused. You cannot change what happened to the child, but it is possible to find this needy child within yourself and to understand and care for him or her in the same way that you might care for any child who is feeling frightened, vulnerable or distressed. With this care, the needy inner child can mature into a strong and independent adult. Without this care, part of you will remain frozen as a needy child who feels frightened and alone. Penny Parks' book *Rescuing the 'Inner Child'* explains these ideas in detail and is well worth reading (see 'Further reading'). Below we suggest two exercises to help you contact and accept your inner child.

Exercise 1: Photograph

Find a photograph of yourself at the age you were being abused. Try to recall what you were like and what you did and felt. Try to remember what emotions you had that you were not able to express, and the times you were misunderstood and not cared for. What kind of love and care did you want that you weren't getting at that time? Keep this photograph with you, and every time you look at it, try to accept the child you were.

Exercise 2: Letter to and from the inner child

Write a letter to this inner child from the adult you are now, allowing yourself to express all the feelings you have towards him or her, both good and bad. Write your letter in simple language, the sort of language a child could understand. Next write a reply from this child to yourself as you are now. Write about how you felt and what you needed that you didn't get. Continue writing letters to and from the inner child until the adult part of yourself is able to support and accept the inner child, and the inner child feels comforted.

This exercise may be much harder to do than it appears, especially for survivors who hate or fear their inner child. You may find yourself feeling upset or disturbed as you begin to experience the pain of your childhood. Take your time. You may need to write a series of letters over a number of weeks or months.

Here are extracts from Luke's letters to and from himself as a child:

Hi,
I want to talk to you about rights. The rights of every person, man, woman or child, black or white, old or young, rich or poor. We have the right to breathe, eat, sleep, play or even go to the toilet. Children and young people especially have the right to be safe yet sometimes their rights are taken away. The right to be safe includes what happens to your body. If someone tries to touch you in a way you don't like you have the right to tell them to stop. It doesn't matter if they are young or old or if they are family members. If you need help, then I am always there. Love, Big Luke

Hi,
Thanks for the letter, no one has ever talked to me like that before, like I matter. You talked about rights, I don't think Mum and Dad think kids have rights. When the abuser touched my penis he wouldn't stop and I couldn't tell him to stop. He was older and I was the youngest and no one listened to me. When he touched me and I enjoyed it I thought it was my fault. Luke

Hi,
Thanks for writing back. You made me feel proud, it takes a lot of courage to talk about the things that happened to you. I respect you and I respect the trust you put in me. I want to tell you that

you do matter and you are worth something. When the abuser touched your penis, he violated your rights. Enjoying the touch was normal. Yet you had nothing to feel ashamed about – he was responsible. I want to talk to you about 'good touch' and 'bad touch'. Good touch is when you get a hug or a kiss that makes you feel safe and loved. Bad touch is when you don't feel safe and feel awkward and uncomfortable. When someone touches you, even if it is someone you love, and you don't like it you are allowed to say 'no', or ask for help. It is your body and your right. Love, Big Luke

Hi,
I don't feel so alone now. It's like I've got a friend, someone who loves me for me. Thank you. Luke

Ingrid's letter was written at a time when she had begun to love and support her inner child.

My dearest Ingrid,
I am sorry you had to wait such a long time on your own, confused and lonely. I did not know you were there and when I first saw you in my mind a few weeks ago, still waiting, still crying, I was frightened and needed to think for a while before making contact with you. Please don't feel sad any more. I am here now, strong enough for both of us. Let me explain to you about what happened. I can still sense your confusion.

As I write now I am looking at a photo of you. You are in a park with mother and your brother, Hans. I picked this photo out because it showed me clearly the difference in size, and consequently power, between you and Hans. It is obvious that you couldn't have stopped him abusing you. Try to remember this. It will help you to stop blaming yourself.

Sometimes you cried during the abuse. You were so young then that you did not know what he was doing but you felt disgusted. What he tried to do with you was something too advanced for your age, something adults do and then it is OK; it is not disgusting when it happens between loving adults. Please, don't be ashamed that you allowed him to touch you and kiss you. You were so eager to be liked by everyone that you were willing to do just about anything in return. Please don't feel bad about this. You have done nothing wrong. Maybe it will help you if you understand why your need to please was so great.

Mother tried to kill herself when you were 2 years old. Father wanted to divorce her. She refused and he stayed but hardly talked to any of the family after that. Mother was so involved in her own problems that she could not see your problems and only looked after your physical needs. Every member of the family was so wrapped up in their own problems that they couldn't give you the love and attention you so desperately needed. It was not because you were not nice enough, it was simply because they needed all their strength to cope with themselves. You thought if you were nicer, more giving and the best at school, they would love you and notice you. You obeyed every wish they had and tried your hardest to please them.

Dearest child, I am on your side, and I will always be standing by you. Nobody has the right to abuse another person, no matter what has happened to them. Hans had no right to do that to you. What you must understand is that the abuse happened because of something in him that made him want to abuse you, not because of anything you did or said. It was his fault the abuse started, his fault it carried on and his responsibility alone. You were only abused because you had to share his bedroom. If another child had been sleeping in that room, that other child would have been abused.

I have learned that it is never too late to change. Just because you have been alone and lonely for almost 40 years, it does not mean you have to stay like that. When I first saw you as the distressed child still within me, I saw you with your arms outstretched, tears streaming down your face and so much in need of love that I cried. I felt bad because you were so unhappy, and because I had neglected you. All we can do now is make a new beginning.

Promise me that you will tell me whenever something frightens or worries you and I will promise you to listen. I will be there for you whenever you need me. You are safe now, and I will make sure that nobody ever hurts you again. Put your hand in mine and come with me. I am your best friend and the one person that will never leave you. I love you, my child. You will never be alone again. Ingrid

Writing the letters to and from the inner child and keeping the photograph of yourself as a child with you, will help you to accept and care for yourself as a child. Once your own inner child feels supported and cared for, you will be better prepared to offer the same support and care to any children and young people you are with.

CONFIDENT PARENTING

You may already have good parenting skills but lack self-confidence. No parent or child is perfect. Tantrums, bedwetting and arguments about eating or bedtime are common at certain ages and do not necessarily mean that you lack skills as a parent. Survivors often begin to feel more confident about their parenting skills once they start to talk with other parents and share their anxieties, problems and different coping methods.

Reading a book on childcare, attending a parenting skills class or talking to someone who is skilled at relating to children, such as a health visitor or teacher, can be useful. Don't be afraid to ask for help or to share your anxieties with others. It is only concerned parents who ask for advice. You can also build up your parenting skills and become more confident by learning to be assertive with your children and discovering useful ways to protect them. We discuss this below.

ASSERTION

Building up self-esteem and self-confidence and learning to behave more assertively can help you feel stronger and more in control of yourself and your children. It can also help you deal more fairly and equally with children and young people. What children feel and want is important, but what you feel and want is important too. Children need to be taught to respect other people's rights as well as their own. Look back at the section on assertion in Chapter 9.

Children are always trying to test out the limits of what they are allowed to do. If you never say 'No', or always allow children to do anything they want, and then suddenly become very angry and restrictive, the children will feel confused. Try using a five-stage system to signal to a child that they are pushing the limits with their behaviour. Start with a simple request and if the child does not do as you ask, 'step up the gears' and become firmer at each stage.

Example of the five-stage system

1 (*Firm voice at normal level*) 'Please don't touch that. It could easily break. Come and look at this.' (*Offer an alternative toy*)
2 (*Firm voice, frown and point at the object*) 'I have told you before, don't touch that. Come away.'

3 (*Raising voice*) 'No! Don't touch.' (*Softer voice, smiling*) 'Come and
   look at this.'
4 (*Keeping voice raised*) 'No! Don't touch that. If you try to do that
   again you will have to go to your bedroom for 5 minutes.' (Or 'I
   will take you home', 'You will not go swimming this afternoon',
   and so on)
5 Carry out what you said you would do at stage 4.

At stage 4, make sure that what you say you will do is not too harsh
or out of proportion to the child's bad behaviour, and that you are
prepared to carry it out. Your child will begin to learn when he or
she is going too far and stop before stage 5. This system also helps
you know what to do next. You can use this method to ask the child
to do something or to stop doing something. If the child is endan-
gering him- or herself, you will, however, need to take immediate
action.

Not being firm and never saying 'No' is exhausting. It will not
help children learn how to deal with other people, nor will it make
them love and respect you. Adults and children respect and like
people who behave assertively rather than allowing themselves to
be walked over. Finding the right balance between what you need
and what the child needs will benefit you both. Children are likely
to grow up feeling self-confident and cared for if they are treated
fairly, consistently and with love.

PROTECTING CHILDREN APPROPRIATELY
Feeling constantly fearful that your children might be abused
comes from feelings of fear and vulnerability resulting from your
own abuse. It is therefore important to sort out your own feelings
first and then work together with your children to help protect
them from abuse. However, you should take immediate action to
keep children and young people away from anyone who has abused
a child. Chapter 16, 'Working towards prevention', looks at how to
protect children and young people from sexual abuse and suggests
a number of guidelines. There are many resources with support and
information about child protection – see 'Sources of help' at the
back of the book.

Survivors may have heard that people who have been sexually
abused become abusers. This is sometimes said but it is not correct.

It is true that some abusers have been sexually abused themselves as children, but most people who have been sexually abused would never abuse children.

Hugging, kissing, stroking and bathing a child are all normal expressions of love and care if they are given and received in that spirit. The same actions can be abusive if they are done for the adult's benefit and are inappropriate or unwanted by the child. **People who are touching children and young people in this way, or are having sexual fantasies about children and young people, need to get help immediately by contacting Stop it Now! (at: <www.stopitnow.org.uk>).**

Learning new and more appropriate ways to protect children can help increase your confidence and remind you that it is not the child's behaviour, dress or words that 'provoke' abuse. It can also help you to feel better about giving your children the affection and love they need.

GETTING HELP FOR YOUR CHILDREN

> I got a social worker and Sarah started a day-nursery full time. The staff would often say that she just sat in a corner playing with a doll. How did I feel about that? I had created this baby and I could not give her what she needed. I felt so bad about it all. Now Sarah is a lot better. She is able to mix with other children and play. With the help we have received, Sarah and I now have a pretty good mother and daughter relationship. **Sally**

If your problems with your children have been going on for a long time, especially if you have been angry and rejecting towards them, they may have developed their own problems and require help. If your child is showing disturbed behaviour or is withdrawn and unhappy, get help for her or him now (see 'Sources of help'). This does not mean you have failed as a parent. It is an acknowledgement of your own problems, and a responsible and caring way to help your child.

Summary

Survivors often have problems relating to children because of the effects of the sexual abuse they experienced themselves when children. As Fiona's story at the start of the chapter shows, this can be overcome with the right sort of help. Working on your memories and feelings about your own sexual abuse, and on your neediness, will allow you to begin to relate to children in their own right rather than as reminders of yourself as a child. Learning new parenting skills will also help you become a better and more confident parent.

After attending a survivors' group, Pam had a very different attitude towards her son.

> I am now aware that my son is a person in his own right and is influenced by his parents, including me. Now I can love my son for the first time and it's wonderful. The things I've missed out on are unbelievable. I wish I'd sought help earlier. It's brilliant to be able to cuddle him, climb into bed with him to read him a bedtime story and to do these things because I love him, not because of a sense of duty. The only thing I can't do yet, because he is a boy, is bathe him, but this is a small problem compared with how I was before. At least he knows I love him and he loves me. **Pam**

It is possible to make things better for you and your children. Keep working on it and don't give up hope.

Suggestions

- Your own history of sexual abuse can affect the way you relate to your own children. Write down any ways in which you think your abuse may have affected the way you feel about, or behave towards, your children. Look at Box 9 and tick off any of the difficulties in relating to children that apply to you.
- The majority of survivors would never harm a child, but some do get sexually aroused by children or have an urge to abuse a child. **If you have any sexual feelings or desires about children, or have touched a child inappropriately, you must seek help for yourself as soon as possible.** Contact Stop it Now! (at: <www.stopitnow.org.uk>) or telephone the NSPCC (0808 800 5000) and see 'Sources of help' at the back of the book.
- You can help yourself to overcome your difficulties in relation to children by learning to become a more confident parent, and

by dealing with your memories and feelings about the abuse and your own neediness. Follow the suggestions and do the exercises described in the chapter.

- There is more information on protecting children and young people from abuse in Chapter 16, 'Working towards prevention'. Talk to your children about how to keep themselves safe, or work through a book about keeping safe with them. Contact one of the resources (for example, NSPCC or Kidscape) in the 'Sources of help'.

- The chapter on 'Childhood' in the *Breaking Free Workbook* contains some exercises that may be useful to you.

13

Mothers

Survivors of sexual abuse often have difficulties in their relationships with their mothers. Mothers are supposed to love, support and protect their children. They are expected to prevent bad things from happening to their children and always be there to listen and to make things better. Children who have been sexually abused have not had this help and protection. They may not have been listened to, and they may not have had a mother there to protect them when needed. In addition, mothers *do* sometimes sexually abuse their children and young people; if this happened to you, work on your relationship with her using Chapter 14, 'Abusers'. More often, however, the mother is not abusing her child and is potentially in a position to help and support the abused child.

In this chapter, we look at the ways in which sexual abuse can affect a survivor's relationship with his or her mother, or a person in a similar caregiving role (this could be a non-abusing father, grandparents or foster parents). Difficulties between mothers and survivors are not inevitable. The mother may realize that her child is being sexually abused and support and protect him or her. The mother–child relationship can be strengthened if the child can share his or her emotions and feel loved and supported.

> My mother found out about the abuse when she heard me cry out from my bedroom and came to investigate. I told her everything that had been going on and her reaction was very positive. She told my father and brother and they got my abuser to leave the house immediately. **Anthony**

Unfortunately, this rarely happens. Mothers usually do not know that their children are being sexually abused, because sexual abuse happens in secret and the child is manipulated to keep the secret. Sometimes mothers do know, or suspect, that their son or daughter is being sexually abused, but do not stop the abuse or protect the child. Mothers may be unable to cope with their own feelings of anger or distress about the abuse of their son or daughter.

213

There are many ways in which sexual abuse can damage, rather than strengthen, the relationship between the child or adult survivor and his or her mother. Survivors' feelings towards their mothers are often a confused mixture of anger, love, hatred, pity, resentment and a desire to protect them. Some of the difficulties survivors experience in their relationships with their mothers are discussed in more detail below. Exercises are suggested to help understand and come to terms with the emotions and overcome the difficulties.

Difficulties with mothers

FEELING PROTECTIVE

> As a child, I felt that telling about the abuse would make my mum more unhappy and she'd feel guilty. I felt very protective towards my mum. **Jane**

Few children and young people tell their mothers that they are being sexually abused. They are frightened of the consequences of telling – of being blamed, disbelieved or punished. Many sexually abused children fear the distress and pain their mothers might feel if they knew what was happening. Abusers often keep children and young people silent by telling them that their mothers would be upset if they knew. Children therefore tolerate great pain themselves in order to protect their mothers. Children find themselves protecting their mothers rather than being protected by them.

> As I got older I didn't want my mum to be upset. How could I hurt her by telling her what had happened? I feel really sorry for her because her life has been so unhappy. I wouldn't like her to feel upset because she didn't protect me. I love her and wish I could change her life for her. **Kate**

Children may feel especially protective if the abuser is the mother's partner. The secrecy can create a barrier between mother and child, and cause difficulties in the relationship between them. The mother cannot understand why her child is distressed or why the child is behaving differently and cannot tell her why.

Many survivors describe having had a close relationship with their mothers until the abuse started. New stepfathers are sometimes jealous of the mother's relationship with her child; abusing the child can have the added 'benefit' for him of destroying this close relationship.

The secrecy frequently continues into adulthood. Survivors who have overcome many of their difficulties and speak openly about their abuse may still be adamant that their mothers must never know. They find it hard to break the habit of protecting their mothers and may look after the mothers' feelings at the expense of their own.

Survivors are often trying to give their mothers the care and protection they would like to have had themselves when they were children. Underlying this caring and giving, however, is often a great well of neediness. Survivors may feel a sense of grief and anger that they never really experienced the feeling of being mothered, and of being dependent and secure, when children; and that as adults they still do not have a close, confiding and trusting relationship with their mothers.

Katarina decided it was better to believe that her mother would have protected her if she had known, rather than tell her and risk a different reaction.

> I could not tell my mother about the abuse. I was frightened what her reactions would be. As long as she didn't know I could cling to the thought she would have protected me. She was a very strong believer in family unity. What if she had not completely separated me from my brother (the abuser)? He would have carried out his threats without doubt and she was too gullible to think bad of her own son. I would have lost that last ray of hope – the complete trust in my mother. **Katarina**

Katarina was not only protecting her mother by not telling; she was also protecting her own hope that if her mother had known she would have given her all the love and protection she needed.

For adult survivors, protecting their mother can create practical problems and add further strain to the relationship. Survivors may find themselves caught up in a web of lies, in an attempt to explain why they are avoiding the abuser or why they are receiving counselling. If the abuser lives with the survivor's mother, the survivor may visit infrequently and keep any children away in order to protect them. Mothers who do not know about the abuse, and do not understand why this is happening, usually feel hurt and rejected by this behaviour.

> I finally decided I never wanted to see my abuser again; so if I knew my brother was visiting my mother, I left before he arrived or didn't go in the first place. I stopped going to her birthday parties or for Christmas dinners. She felt very hurt by this and often asked me why. I told her it was because I didn't like my brother but when asked for the reason, I remained silent. She asked my brother. He told her he didn't know what I could have against him, he hadn't done anything wrong. She was very hurt by my behaviour but I thought she would feel even more hurt if she knew the truth. She could blame me for being wilful; if she had known the truth she would have blamed herself. **Katarina**

Survivors may jeopardize their own relationships with their mothers in order to protect them from knowing about the abuse.

FEELING NEGLECTED
Survivors often feel angry, upset or resentful about their mother's failure to notice that they were being sexually abused. Mothers are expected to be sensitive to their children's feelings and needs, and to know what is happening to them. When children's distress is not noticed, children may feel let down and neglected, even if they have consciously tried to hide the abuse from their mothers and put on a cheerful front. Jane felt let down by her mother's failure to make time for her and really listen and find out what was wrong.

> I was abused by my stepfather from the age of about 7 to 17. My mother's marriage to my father had been a violent one and that's why she divorced him. My mother worked hard, studying to become a teacher. When she married my stepfather we moved to Wakefield. I don't think she suspected that he was abusing me and my sister Lizzie. If we had nightmares or tantrums, she thought we were disturbed because of the access visits with our father.
> The more I look back over my childhood the more I realize how absent she was. I used to think she threw herself into her work (teaching) because she was unhappy at home, in her marriage. I didn't feel that my mother was there for me. With

hindsight I can understand why, but at the time it made me feel that I was not worth being looked after. **Jane**

Many survivors feel angry with their mothers for not noticing the abuse. Katarina feels her mother should have realized that she was being abused.

> I was 4 or 5 years old when my brother ejaculated between my closed legs. His semen wet my nightclothes and the sheet. I was blamed for wetting the bed. As an adult now I feel a mixture of anger and contempt for my mother for not noticing the difference between semen and urine when she changed my nightclothes and sheet. **Katarina**

If the abuse remains secret and these feelings from childhood are not resolved, adult survivors may continue to feel let down and uncared for in their relationships with their mothers, whatever their mothers do. They continue to silently hope that their mothers will notice their distress and voluntarily offer the care and support they crave. When this does not happen, survivors may be over-whelmed with anger and distress, and emotionally withdraw from their mothers in an attempt to protect themselves and to punish their mothers.

FEELING ABANDONED AND BADLY TREATED
In some cases, mothers are aware that abuse is happening and take no action to stop it. They accuse the children of lying or turn a blind eye to it and allow the children to continue to be abused.

> When I finally told my mum about being abused by my dad and by her boyfriend, she said I had made it all up. As far back as I can remember my mum would try to convince me that things I knew to be true, were lies; and in the end I would just believe her. At one point, I tried to convince myself that perhaps I had dreamt it all. I know she knew about it though, even before I said anything, because I can remember hearing her and her boyfriend arguing about it. **Sally**

Some mothers support and stay with abusive partners, even if this means losing custody of their children or destroying their relation-ship with the adult survivors. As an adult, Joanne told her mother she had been abused by her stepfather, Ken, and was then blamed and abandoned by her. Her mother chose to stay with Ken, even though he had just been released from prison for abusing his biological daughter.

> I felt hurt at my mother's decision to side with my stepfather and abandon my family and me for him. **Joanne**

Even if mothers stop the abuse or leave the abuser, they may still be angry at the survivors or blame them for what has happened. Some mothers are openly hostile and treat the survivors badly. Others are cold and distant and play on the survivors' feelings of guilt. The adult survivors may feel angry and resentful towards their mothers for abandoning them and treating them badly. They may find ways to get back at their mothers or feel consumed with a rage they cannot express. However, survivors are often devastated by their mothers' reactions and feel no anger but an enormous sense of grief and loss.

> I still feel very confused about my mother. Although I am the victim, I am the one who has lost my family. I now don't speak to any of my family except my auntie. I don't know what hurts the most – the abuse or losing my family because of it all. I have a husband, three smashing kids and a nice home but I still wish I had a proper mum and a grandma for my kids. **Sally**

They may try to gain their mothers' love and understanding by doing things for them and always trying to please them.

> I have always had a bad relationship with my mum. I have tried hundreds of times to make it better but the more I tried, and the more I did for her, the more she wanted and thus the relationship was one-sided. On the few occasions she did anything to help me, I never seemed to be able to show her enough thanks. **Sally**

Some survivors continue to accept poor treatment from their mothers, or continue to be abused and disregarded by them, in the hope of one day gaining the love and acceptance they crave. Others, like Sally, may stop seeing their mothers but continue to feel abandoned and grieve for the loss of the relationship.

DEALING WITH MOTHERS' DISTRESS ABOUT THE ABUSE

> There are really no words to describe my feelings when I understood that my daughters had been sexually abused. It was something like hearing of the death of someone you love – in

fact, something did die. There was pain and an overwhelming sense of loss and desperation. When that passed there was overwhelming anger. Anger against my husband for his treachery and against the girls for what seemed like deceit on their part because they had not told me. I was angry with God that such evil had overtaken us. I had a tremendous feeling of failure which crept into all my activities and sapped my self-confidence. I swung between thoughts of murder and suicide but ended up rejecting both. **Grace (Jane's mother)**

Mothers are often thrown into emotional turmoil when they find out that their daughter or son has been sexually abused. They may be overwhelmed by grief, anger, distress or feelings of failure and helplessness. They may also suffer financial and practical problems if the disclosure results in a marriage break-up or a breadwinner going to prison. Survivors can have great difficulty in coping with their mothers' distress about the abuse, and this may add to their own feelings of guilt.

My sister Lizzie and I finally decided to tell our mother about the abuse because we felt that it would help her understand the estranged relationship between her and Lizzie. When we told her, I didn't doubt that she believed us, but she was very upset, as I had always imagined she would be. I felt responsible for causing her that pain and distress. We didn't discuss our feelings or any details about the abuse with her. I really felt that she couldn't cope with any more. **Jane**

Survivors often blame themselves for causing their mothers' distress, and other people may also blame them for disclosing the abuse. Some mothers openly express their distress. Mothers may look to their son or daughter for support, especially if the abuse has remained a secret between the two of them, but survivors may feel unable to cope with their mothers' feelings as well as their own emotional pain. Mothers and survivors thrown together in this situation often cannot help each other and may make each other's problems worse. Survivors may also feel that their mothers are so involved with their own distress that the survivors' feelings and needs are being overlooked (again).

My mother would not be honest with me in discussions and always turned it round to discussing her own unhappy childhood. Perhaps this was her way of coping with her guilty feelings but I began to feel strongly that I could no longer rationalize or cope with her feelings when I was trying to help myself. **Jane**

Survivors may find themselves in the familiar position of trying to protect, support and 'mother' their own mothers, and they feel angry and resentful about the situation.

Alternatively, both mothers and their son or daughter may avoid mentioning the sexual abuse or the abuser, for fear of upsetting the other person. This creates a barrier between them and may lead to misunderstandings and a lack of closeness in the relationship. Melanie thought she had ruined her parents' lives by disclosing the abuse. She did not talk about the abuse again because she felt guilty and didn't want to hurt her mother.

> Mum never knew exactly what did happen to me. I could never really talk about it. I felt I had broken my mum and dad up as a normal husband and wife, as from that time on my mother didn't want anything to do with him on the sexual side of the marriage. What happened to me turned her right off. She blamed my dad as he was nearby when it was happening. **Melanie**

Melanie's mother, however, felt guilty for not protecting her daughter. She thought Melanie blamed her and so she avoided mentioning the abuse. The relationship became more and more strained, and they both became extremely sensitive to any criticism from each other.

Dealing with the difficulties

Below we look at ways in which you can begin to explore and understand your feelings towards your mother, and consider what changes you might make in your relationship. Dealing with the general problems caused by your sexual abuse by working through this book and by talking to other survivors or a counsellor can also help. It is useful to read this section and do the exercises even if your mother is dead or if you have no contact with her.

EXPLORING YOUR FEELINGS

The relationship between you and your mother may involve many complex and conflicting feelings. You may not have allowed yourself time to find out what you really feel about your mother. As an abused child, you may have felt that your feelings did not matter and that you had no right to express them. It is useful to get in touch with these childhood feelings by doing the letter-writing exercise from the inner child (see Chapter 12) before going on to the exercise below.

This exercise helps you to explore your feelings towards your mother and express them in a safe way. You may be surprised by your feelings. Many survivors think they feel only anger for their mothers, but discover that underneath they yearn to be loved and accepted. Others find that the love and respect they feel towards their mother masks strong feelings of anger and resentment.

Exercise: Letter to your mother
Write a letter to your mother (not to send) expressing all the feelings you have towards her and all the things you would never dare say. The letter could be hand-written or typed into your computer or other device. Below are four examples of letters written by survivors.

Joanne's letter

Dear Mother,
It's sad when you realize a mother and daughter relationship is over, even if it wasn't very good to begin with. I remember the letter you wrote to me after you heard that I was going to the police. 'How could you do this to me?,' you said. How could I cause you to be by yourself if he were to be convicted once more? I'm afraid I was so full of anger at the time that that point didn't come into it.

I know that the day I brought the abuse out into the open with you was the final straw and after that we seemed to drift apart for ever. You asked why we didn't visit with the children when Ken was in the house. I never said at the time that I could remember the time you came home early to find the doors locked while I was being abused; and the day I was trying to tell you what he was doing to me only to remember his threats and back down, afraid to finish the sentence. I never said I could remember the time you shoved a newspaper article under his nose on a case of incest and took no further action when he just laughed off the suggestion and said you were being stupid. Why on earth didn't you protect me from his abuse? Indeed, why didn't you protect yourself, me and my brothers from his cruelty and violence? I feel even more hurt that you didn't protect us now that I have children of my own. What kind of a mother were you?

I know you probably cannot understand why I am still so bitter at what Ken did to me. Perhaps you believe that because the abuse has ended I shouldn't still be affected by it. What a misconception that is. Though perhaps you could be excused for thinking that, as even I had no idea that the abuse was the cause of all my current problems until I began meeting with the survivors' group.

Now I'm really glad that I have had the opportunity to air my feelings with you. They have haunted me for years. It does sound sad but it looks likely that my life will continue without you. How sad it is that we couldn't have a close relationship with one another as I believe every mother and child should have, but you have made your choice, mother, and decided to stand by the man who sexually abused his daughter and indeed your own daughter. How can I ever come to terms with that?

Polly's letter

Dear Mum,

I am writing this down as I found it hard to say. I want to tell you how I feel and have felt over the years. When I confronted you about Grandad you said we had to understand that my nanna was a cold person and that my grandad was a sensitive warm person. This was your excuse for what he did to us. Well, I think that is rubbish. If he needed sex that much then why didn't he find a prostitute or leave nanna, but to abuse us children was wrong. I feel angry at you because you didn't protect us in spite of it happening to you when you were little. You say he put his hands down your pants but you told him not to and he stopped. Well, he did worse things to us. He made us have anal sex, oral sex, made us touch his penis and do other things.

Why is it that none of us could talk to you? You were so strict about anything to do with sex, like turning TV channels over, never talking about periods or anything. Yet all those years you let that happen to all of us and not only from Grandad but also other men as well. I could scream at you sometimes.

I couldn't understand how you never noticed or did you just ignore it? You keep going on about how wonderful he is. Well, I don't want you to, because it makes me feel sick. He was an old perverted bastard and I hate him. The way you just overlook everything makes me hate you as well. You have always blamed nanna for it all but you are blaming the wrong person. You are trying to put your guilt on to everyone except yourself. You cannot go on burying your head in the sand.

Luke's letter

Dear Mother,
As I try to focus on what I feel about you and the part you played, I realize I love you and still want to protect you. From what? Me and my hatred!

My idea of what a parent should be seems to be the opposite of yours. All you had to do was love us. When I look back I get the feeling we were nothing more than pets. As you read down the page you are probably thinking this is just Luke with a chip on his shoulder but it is not. It's about you leaving me unprotected so that vile filthy bastard could do what the fuck he liked to me. Surely even you could see that it is a mother's role to protect her children. Didn't you at least cotton on when he was caught with my brother? Do you remember what you said to me? 'Don't do anything you shouldn't.' My God, how many 11-year-olds could stop a manipulating sly cunning bastard like that? You know from that moment on you walked away from me. I was so lonely. I felt so dirty, so ashamed and had to keep the secret.

You have done me no favours. I have nothing to thank you for, you failed me, you let me down. I want to walk out of your life and never have to enter it again. I despise you and dislike you with great intensity, yet I still love you. My life is getting increasingly better, no thanks to you. When you see me with my wife and kids, it's no thanks to you. For your sake, you won't get this letter. See how your perfect loving son still protects you!

Lorna's letter

Dear Mum,
I want to know why you didn't help me when Uncle Sam was abusing me. Why didn't you know? Why didn't you stop him? There were lots of times I wanted to tell you what was going on but you never seemed to be there for long enough and anyway I didn't think you cared. Even when you thought I had run away you just punished me. Why didn't it occur to you that I was frightened? I know you thought I did not care about you as much as my brothers and sisters did. I did but I just didn't know how to let you know. There were times I hated you because you didn't

help me. Sometimes I felt like screaming at you that I was there and I needed you as much as the others. It seemed that you did not care or you were too busy to notice, I don't know which.

Notice if you are directing all your anger for the abuse towards your mother and excusing the abuser. Mothers are not responsible for abuse committed by another person. Mothers who fail to listen to the child, to take action or to stop the abuse are responsible for this, but the abuser is always responsible for the sexual abuse itself. Many survivors initially blame themselves for the abuse, then move on to blaming their mothers for not protecting them, and then finally place the responsibility for the abuse with the perpetrator.

Exercise: Letter from your mother

If you have already written a letter to your mother, you can now write a reply to that letter. Write a letter to yourself *as if you were your mother*, at the time you were being abused. Seeing the situation through your mother's eyes can help you understand that your mother may not have known about the abuse. Until recent years, most mothers were not aware of the risk to their children and young people of sexual abuse, especially from relatives or friends. If you were behaving badly or strangely *because of the abuse*, the idea that you were being sexually abused would probably never have occurred to your mother.

Seeing the situation through your mother's eyes can also help you understand that she treated you the way she did because of her own circumstances, not because you were a bad or unlovable child. She may have been too busy to notice your distress, or unable to cope with the circumstances she was in. She may have been afraid of losing her partner, her home, her family. She may have been depressed, anxious, angry or resentful about her own life, or she may have been sexually abused herself.

Mothers may cope with the suspicion that their child is being sexually abused by pushing it to the back of their minds, blocking it out and pretending it isn't happening. They may remain silent because they fear the consequences of telling. Whatever your mother's problems or circumstances, she was still responsible if she neglected you, treated you badly or abandoned you. The aim of this letter-writing exercise is not to make excuses for your mother's behaviour. It is to help you understand that you did deserve love and protection. She behaved the way she did because this was her way of dealing with life and not because you were unlovable.

Lorna wondered if she hadn't been protected because her mother didn't care. However, when she thought about the family circumstances at the time she was being abused, she realized her mother was trying to cope with working night shifts, a husband who was always out drinking, and bringing up six children (one of whom was in hospital). Lorna then wrote this reply to herself from her mother.

> Dear Lorna,
> I could not help you when your Uncle Sam was abusing you because I did not know what he was doing. I knew that you didn't like him but you would not say why. I asked you lots of times but you just pulled the shutters down on me. There were times I tried to talk to you or listen to you, but you were not having any of it. It's true that I punished you when I thought you had run away but I did not know what else I could do. You would not, or could not, talk to me. I thought you were playing me up. Your sister was in hospital and I had four other children at home to look after besides you. There was not always the time that was needed for everyone. All my children had been fairly happy, then you changed and became moody and would not talk to me. It was really difficult. I knew you were unhappy but I could not help you because I did not know how to. I also had other responsibilities. I thought I had lost you but I did not know what I had done wrong or what I could do to help you.

Lorna realized that, although her mother had failed to protect her, it was because of the family's circumstances and because her mother did not know how to help, not because Lorna was unlovable. You may find yourself feeling less angry with your mother as you begin to understand her situation more, or cease to blame her for things she was not responsible for. You may find yourself feeling angry with her for the first time, because you realize you have been protecting your mother when she should have been protecting you.

MAKING CHANGES
Relationships between mothers and their sons or daughters are never perfect. Many difficulties can arise that are nothing to do

with sexual abuse. Mothers are never able to live up to the image of the ideal mother, and children invariably feel hurt in some way by their parents. It is realistic to accept that there may be some difficulties. You may never have the totally loving and supportive mother you would really like. Being frequently upset, damaged or abused by your mother is, however, not acceptable.

Many survivors feel that they cannot assert themselves with their mothers, and feel themselves to be victims of their mothers' putdowns, constant demands, lack of support or insensitive treatment. Like Sally's mother, your mother may have convinced you that you are always in the wrong. Remember that, as an abused child, you became accustomed to being treated badly, without respect and as if your feelings and needs did not matter. You may have learnt to put up with this type of behaviour and accepted it. Survivors may also continue to accept bad treatment from their mothers because they feel:

- powerless to do anything else;
- frightened of having an argument;
- frightened of losing the relationship;
- that they deserve to be treated badly;
- that they are useless, no good or to blame for being abused;
- that they are in the wrong or being unreasonable;
- that they have to respect their mothers and do as they are told;
- that they have to try to please them;
- that they are to blame for upsetting them/making them angry;
- that they are to blame for breaking up the family;
- that their own feelings are not as important as other people's.

No one deserves to be treated badly. Both you and your mother are adults and could have an equal relationship where you respect your own and each other's rights. Accept that there may be difficulties, but don't accept being used and abused. Passively accepting bad treatment, and trying desperately to please, will not gain your mother's love, as Sally discovered. Ask yourself if this approach has worked so far.

Feeling less guilty and responsible for the abuse, and for your mother's feelings, can help you feel and behave differently. You may be able to make changes in the relationship with your mother by changing your behaviour, discussing the problems and requesting that she makes changes in her behaviour. Talking openly and honestly is a good way to encourage someone else to do the same. Behaving assertively encourages other people to behave assertively in return and discourages abusive behaviour. Working through the following exercises can be helpful even if you decide not to confront your mother face to face.

Exercise 1
Write a description of the relationship you have with your mother. Think about the way she treats you and the way you treat her. What do you like about the relationship? What do you dislike? Is the relationship with your mother good for you, or are you being damaged and abused?

Exercise 2
Make a list of some of the things you would like to change with your mother, starting with the easiest items first.

Example

1 I want to ask her to come to my house once a fortnight instead of me always going to her house.
2 I want to say 'No' to going to Sunday dinner every week.
3 I want to ask her not to give the children presents every time she sees them.
4 I want to tell her that I feel hurt and upset when she criticizes my appearance and ask her not to do it.
5 I want to tell her that I don't want to hear about what a wonderful man her father (my abuser) was.

Pick out the easiest task from your list and write down how you might approach this assertively with your mother. Decide what you want to say and how you can say it assertively. Write down all the different ways in which your mother might react and how you could respond. Get a friend to pretend to be your mother and practise what you could say. Speak to your mother only if you want to, and after you have done this practice and feel confident.

TALKING TO YOUR MOTHER ABOUT THE ABUSE
You may want to tell your mother about the abuse or, if she already knows, to talk to her about it again. This can help the relationship

by breaking the silence, clearing up any misunderstandings and allowing each of you to express your feelings. However, this may not be a helpful step to take. You need to use your own judgement and talk it over with a friend or a professional helper. Telling your mother is not an essential part of the healing process, and you may decide you do not want to do this. If you do decide to disclose to your mother, make sure you only do so after careful preparation, and when you are quite sure that you know you are not to blame for what happened. Read the section in Chapter 14 on regaining your power from the abuser.

The preparations you need to make before disclosing to your mother are very similar. Prepare yourself for all the different reactions your mother might have – for example, being upset, angry, not believing you. Act out what might happen, with someone else playing the part of your mother, so you can rehearse your responses. If possible, arrange for both your mother and yourself to have someone around to support you afterwards. Be prepared for the fact that things will not be better immediately, but it may help in the long term.

If the abuse is already known to your mother, there may be more talking that needs to be done. Twenty years after Melanie had first told her mother about the abuse, she brought up the subject again and they were able to clear up their misunderstandings and develop a better relationship.

> Since the abuse, the relationship between my mother and myself had been very strained. A while ago I did manage to talk to her about it. It seemed to help us both to form a closer knit relationship. It was very hard to talk to her about it but afterwards we seemed to communicate better. **Melanie**

Melanie realized she wasn't to blame for her mother's upset, nor for the difficulties in the relationship between her parents. The survivor is not responsible for his or her mother's distress. It is the abuser, by his or her actions, who is responsible for causing distress to the survivor and to the survivor's mother.

> Since I received both one-to-one therapy and group therapy, I don't feel responsible for the abuse any more. My stepfather was responsible. This has also made me feel less responsible for my mother. **Jane**

Survivors can encourage their mothers to get help from a therapist. Jane encouraged her mother, Grace, to have individual therapy. Later Jane, her sister Lizzie and Grace went for therapy together to try to sort out the difficulties they had in relating to each other.

> By the time my mother, my sister and I met together, our mother had had some one-to-one therapy and had had a chance to talk about her feelings in a more constructive situation. I felt that she had had time for reflection. She was less defensive than she had been previously about what my sister and I had to say and I think she really listened. The situation didn't allow her to use diversions as she had done previously. The psychologist was objective and could reflect back what each of us was saying and allow us to clarify what we meant. Also, because the psychologist was there, I felt safe. **Jane**

NOT SEEING YOUR MOTHER

Sometimes it is not possible for survivors to change their relationships with their mothers. A mother who supports the abuser, or blames the survivor for the abuse, may demand that the survivor retracts the disclosure or takes the blame for the abuse. Survivors who are presented with these ultimatums, or have tried to improve their relationship with their mothers and are still being put down, damaged or abused, may decide that the only thing they can do is to stop seeing their mothers. This might be a temporary or permanent solution to the problem.

Sally held on to the relationship with her mother for many years, trying to please her and win her love and support. Sally's mother continued to blame and disbelieve her, turned other family members against her, and tried to cause trouble between Sally and her husband. Sally eventually thought that holding on to the relationship, and the small hope that her mother would change, was not worth all the pain and grief it was causing.

> I always wanted to be able to talk to my mum and tell her how I felt and even to have a good mother and daughter relationship. I know now that it will never be. I have not been in touch with my mum for over a year and now I feel free to get on with my life with my husband and children. **Sally**

Although abandoning a relationship with your mother might be extremely painful, it may be the right choice for you. You do not have to maintain a relationship with anyone just because he or she is a family member. Some survivors choose to distance themselves from their mothers or stop seeing them while they are working through their own problems and resume the relationship when they feel stronger.

Summary

Survivors often have difficulties with their mothers because of the sexual abuse. They may feel neglected, abandoned or badly treated. They may also have a strong desire to protect their mothers from knowing about the abuse or feel responsible for the distress that disclosure can cause. Survivors' feelings towards their mothers may be a mixture of love, hate, resentment, pity, anger and disappointment. Survivors can work on these problems by exploring and expressing their feelings and then trying to make changes in the relationship. In this way, survivors can sort out their feelings towards their mothers, refuse to accept bad treatment, regain their own power and move towards a better relationship.

Suggestion

Follow the suggestions and exercises outlined in the chapter to help you understand your feelings towards your mother and make positive changes. The chapter on 'Mothers' in the *Breaking Free Workbook* contains more detailed exercises to help you understand the difficulties in your relationship with your mother and the feelings you have towards her, and explores why some mothers do not protect their children.

14

Abusers

There were so many years during which I wanted you to like me and have the relationship of 'big brother' that some of my friends had, and that I envied so much. I don't think you ever did like me. There were years in which I hated you so much I thought daily of ways to kill you. **Katarina**

Katarina, in common with many survivors, had conflicting feelings about her abuser. She wanted to have a normal loving brother–sister relationship with him but she also hated him for what he was doing to her. Children and young people usually have negative feelings towards their abusers because of the abuse, but they may also have positive feelings, especially if the abusers are close relatives or friends.

In Chapter 3, we looked at how abusers set up situations where they can manipulate and abuse children and young people, and at some of the reasons why they abuse. In this chapter, we will look at the kinds of people who abuse children, the feelings survivors have towards their abusers, and ways in which these feelings can be explored and expressed.

What are abusers like?

What kinds of people abuse children and young people? Here is a list of some of the characteristics Kate saw in her father.

Cunning, deceitful, a liar, gives the impression he's helpful and generous but this is only to cover the abuse that will follow or because he's afraid someone may tell. Disloyal – uses information told in confidence to suit him. Bad-tempered and violent. Puts others down to elevate himself. Tries to make people feel sorry for him. Thinks his views alone are the right views, he's never wrong. If you disagree or put another view forward you're wrong and shouted down. Selfish. **Kate**

To the outside world, however, he was a respected businessman admired by many.

> This monster robbed me of the first 30 years of my life. Yet no one outside the family suspected. Social workers liked him, educational welfare officers liked him, some teachers liked him, policemen liked him. But they didn't know his secret. **Kate**

Jane's stepfather (her abuser) was cruel and manipulative within the home but gave a very different impression of himself to the local community. An abuser may be seen by outsiders as a good, kind, generous and respected member of the community, the kind of person who looks after others, not the kind of person who would abuse a child. This can be very difficult for the abused children. It can confirm their beliefs that they are to blame for the abuse, and that no one will believe them if they try to tell. Some abusers, like Joanne's, are violent and cruel.

> My stepfather was a violent man and he would drink heavily every night at the pub. He'd come home and beat my mother and us if we got in the way. I remember him hitting my mother so badly that she had to stay in hospital for a week. He was mentally cruel towards us all too. On reflection, I can see he was very immature and took great pleasure in cruelly teasing us. We weren't allowed indoors even when the weather was bad. My brothers and I would stand on the other side of the garden fence and stare into the kitchen window because we were so cold. **Joanne**

Other abusers are quiet, kind and fun to be with. Very few abusers fit the stereotype of a dirty old man. Abusers may be young or old, male or female, rich or poor, kind or cruel, scruffy or smart, strong or frail. Abusers may be dominant men who rule their families with a rod of iron, weak ineffectual men, women who keep themselves to themselves, or friendly young men who are well liked in the neighbourhood. In fact, they are indistinguishable from any other parent, relative, neighbour or friend. Abusers may be labourers, members of parliament, professors, unemployed people, shop-keepers, stockbrokers, social workers, psychologists, taxi drivers, doctors, teachers, football coaches, clergy, celebrities or from *any* other occupation.

Although the majority of abusers are men, women also abuse children (perhaps 14 per cent of the perpetrators of abuse against boys, and 6 per cent against girls, are women). It is difficult for people to accept that women can and do abuse children, especially that women can sexually abuse their own children. It is particularly difficult for victims, both male and female, to accept or disclose that they were abused by women, especially if it was their mother. A mother is supposed to nurture and protect her children, and those children who are abused by their mother may feel they have suffered the greatest betrayal of all.

Accurately identifying what percentage of abusers are female is, however, difficult, especially as victims find it so difficult to talk about abuse by women. Women sexually abuse children and young people on their own, or with a male perpetrator, or sometimes as part of a group of abusers. Graham's mother sexually abused him and his brother, and also allowed other adults from a network of paedophiles to abuse them. It is not possible to tell abusers from non-abusive people unless you know they are sexually abusing children and young people. People of all classes, cultures, religions, ages and personalities can be perpetrators of sexual abuse.

Feelings towards the abuser

> I lie awake at night and I can feel you groping me and I am physically sick. At the memory of your name I'm sick. I could stab you and think I'd done nothing. Torture wouldn't be sufficient punishment for you. I hope when you die you go to hell, but even that's too good for you. I will never ever forgive you for what you've done. You deserve anything evil that comes your way. **Pam**

Pam's feelings towards her abuser (her father) are quite straightforward: she hates him. Kate too is angry at her abuser (her father) for the damage he has done to her and to his many other victims.

> I feel anger that he robbed me of my childhood, stopped me from developing my skills to the full and made me miss opportunities through lack of confidence. I will never, never be able to trust my abuser, even though he may stop abusing. I feel annoyed with him that he's been so disloyal to his wife and family and that he's damaged so many lives. I feel angry that so many people, male and female, have lost years out of their lives because of him. **Kate**

Kate also feels sorry for her abuser.

I pity the abuser, he now has to live with himself and at some stage in his life he surely will have to admit to himself the terrible things he's done and the harm he has caused others. I feel sorry because he must be a sad and lonely man – being an abuser made him miss out on a lot of important relationships in his life. **Kate**

Children are brought up to believe they should love their families, so feel confused when parents, or the people taking care of them, also abuse them. Children may love their fathers, brothers, mothers, sisters, uncles and find it hard to understand how someone they love can hurt them so much. When Sheila first came for therapy, she talked about how much she loved her father even though he had physically and sexually abused her. She blamed herself for the abuse and felt no anger towards him. After she started to under-stand that he was responsible for the abuse, she began to feel angry with him, although she still loved him. This is what she wrote after his death:

Why did you have to leave me? I wish you knew what sort of a mess you have left behind. It's so unfair of you to have escaped the way you did. Believe it or not, there were times when I really loved you and other times when I hated you. I wish you could see the pain that I feel inside. I sometimes sit and think about the past and what you did to me and I feel so hurt and angry. I feel that you have destroyed me inside and that you have taken away part of my life. When I was young I loved and trusted you, and you just used me. How could you do that to me? I will always remember when I was young how I followed you everywhere. You were like some kind of hero to me. I thought I was very special to you, but now when I think of those days I just want to cry for it hurt so much. I felt so guilty when I came up to the hospital to see you the first time you tried to commit suicide. I thought it was my fault because the night before I stood up to you and said 'No' and ran away from you. So, when you came home again I never said anything to you, even though you were hurting me and ruining my childhood, because I did not want you to leave me. I wish things could have been different, for I really did love you. **Sheila**

Abusers can be kind to children and young people and take them on outings, give them treats they would not normally get and pay them a lot of attention. They win the children's trust and affection.

Children may therefore love the abuser and enjoy spending time with him or her, but feel confused when the abuser behaves sexually towards them. Young people may have been groomed to believe the abuser was a boyfriend and they were in a caring relationship.

Moira was abused by her half-brother, Ian, and at times she hated him for the pain she felt because of the abuse. Yet he was her closest friend throughout her childhood and he had loved, protected and comforted her, as well as abusing her.

How can I still love Ian and want to put my arms around him and tell him I still love him and forgive him, and yet in the next breath want to tell him I hate him and want to beat the living daylights out of him? I'm so confused. **Moira**

It can be difficult for a survivor to feel anger towards an abuser whom he or she also loves. Abusers can appear to be warm and caring people when they are not abusing. This can be very confusing for the child, and it strengthens the child's belief that he or she must have done something wrong for the abuser to act like this. The child feels there must be something bad in him or her that brings out this uncharacteristic behaviour in the abuser, and this can make the child turn the anger inwards. This results in young people hating themselves and blaming themselves for the abuse. If a survivor believes he or she is responsible for the abuse, then the perpetrator cannot be to blame for the abuse, so the survivor can keep on loving the abuser.

In adulthood, survivors may continue to love their abusers despite the pain the abuser inflicted on them. Some survivors are so terrified of their abusers that they see them, hear them, smell them or feel their touch when they are not there, and even when the abusers are dead (trauma-based hallucinations). They have been traumatized by the acts and threats used during the abuse and continue to relive parts of the abuse as adults (see the section on hallucinations in Chapter 8).

Survivors experience all sorts of feelings towards their abusers, including hate, love, fear, guilt, concern, disgust, affection, betrayal, pity and anger. They often have a complex mixture of these feelings, which can leave them feeling confused. The exercises below may help you understand and work through your feelings towards the person or persons who abused you.

Working on your feelings about the abuser

Exploring your feelings towards your abuser(s) and finding a way of expressing these feelings can help you break free of your confusion and pain. It can help to talk to a counsellor or therapist about this.

Sometimes it is not helpful to talk to friends and relatives about your abuser as they may feel angry about what has happened to you and expect you to feel angry towards your abuser too.

Polly feels nothing but hate towards her abuser (her grandfather), whereas her sister (who was also abused by him) still loves him. The sisters feel angry with each other because of this difference, and cannot share their feelings or talk about the abuse. Polly believes her sister should also hate her grandfather.

You cannot change your feelings because you or other people think you should. There is no right or wrong way to feel. It is important to begin by recognizing and accepting your feelings for your abuser, whatever they are, and to start to work from there. In therapy, survivors begin to understand that their abusers were responsible for the abuse and that the abusers manipulated the children and young people into the abusive situation. They realize that it is the abuser who is to blame for the abuse and not themselves. For the first time, like Sheila and Moira, they begin to lose their anger at themselves and turn the anger towards their abusers.

As you work through your feelings, you may find that you are also angry at the abuser you believed you loved; or that you love the abuser you thought you only hated; or that under your anger is grief at losing your childhood. The following exercises may help you to discover and release some of your emotions. About 50 per cent of the Wakefield survivors have been sexually abused by more than one person. If you have had more than one abuser, apply the suggestions in this chapter to each of them in turn. Some of the exercises may seem strange to you, so choose one that you feel comfortable with.

Exercise: Talking to a cushion

This exercise can be a useful way for you to explore your own feelings towards your abuser and to express them without having to consider his or her reaction. Do this exercise when you are alone and feeling safe and feel ready to begin to work through your feelings about your abuser.

- Pick a cushion to represent your abuser. Sit on a chair and place the cushion on another chair opposite you, at whatever feels the most comfortable distance.
- Imagine the cushion is your abuser and start to talk to him or her. Begin by telling your abuser how he or she has damaged your life. You may feel many emotions rising in you – accept them and express them to the abuser. Often, talking isn't enough. If you get angry, you may want to throw the cushion on the ground and punch it, stamp on it or kick it around the room. This is a useful way for you to let your feelings out without hurting yourself or anyone else. In fact, this technique is useful whenever you get angry at someone.

Anger is only one of the feelings that may arise. You may feel sadness, fear, love, hate, pity, distaste or any mixture of feelings. The aim of the exercise is to allow you to discover what you are feeling and express your feelings *outwardly*, instead of holding them in or harming yourself. The idea of talking to a cushion may seem strange but many people have really benefited from venting their feelings in this way.

Exercise: Letter to the abuser

Writing a letter to your abuser, without sending it, is another way for you to explore and express your feelings. Allow yourself plenty of time and let yourself write whatever comes into your head. You may want to describe all the things the abuser did to you and how it made you feel at the time. You may want to tell him or her how the abuse affected your life as you grew older, and how you feel towards him or her now.

Writing can help you access the full range of your feelings and give you an opportunity to get them off your chest. It is important that you do this exercise for your own benefit and do not actually send the letter.

Polly's grandfather had abused her and all her sisters. When she was a young adult, Polly had written and posted a letter to her grandfather about the abuse, but when her family found out, they forced her to write again and retract what she had said and apologize to her grandfather. Polly felt betrayed yet again and was left feeling intensely angry. After she had been in a survivors' group,

Polly wanted to confront her grandfather again but he had since died. She wrote another letter to him, this time for herself.

Polly's letter

Dear Bastard,

Yes, Bastard – because you are this and many more names. I confronted you before in a letter telling you I forgive you for everything you did to me. I was made to deny it for my nanna's sake in case she might have a heart attack or something.

I now know that you abused all my sisters and my mum. So it was not a matter of any of us leading you on. You were the guilty one, and you did whatever you wanted to do to innocent children who could not defend themselves and you made them swear to secrecy.

Well, you dirty old pig, it's time you realized what you have done. We could have had you sent to prison for good because there are too many of us for the courts to say it is our imagination. So how does it make you feel to know you are hated intensely by your own grandchildren? Not once did you show any remorse by saying you were sorry, although you had plenty of opportunities. Now you're dead the past has not died with you. I'm so glad you're dead because now I won't have to worry about other children being around a monster like you.

The abuse is not going to ruin my life because I'm fighting it and getting help. People like you are the ones who need help, yet you're that sick you think you're normal. I would hate to be in your shoes because I believe in God, whether you do or not, and you will find punishment for what you've done.

I hope you rot in hell. Polly

After writing this letter, Polly felt she had at last been able to express her true feelings and she began to feel less troubled by her anger.

Anthony was abused by his uncle and as an adult felt very angry towards him. However, every time Anthony saw his uncle, he felt like a frightened young boy again and got away from him as quickly as possible. Writing this letter helped Anthony express his anger and begin to regain his power.

Anthony's letter

If I ever got hold of you I would kill you but maybe that would be too good for you. Can't you see that you have turned my world upside down these past 14 years? What was up with you? Couldn't you get pleasure with someone your own fucking age? All you are is a dirty old man and I hope you will rot in hell. Anthony

Shirley wanted to vent her anger and tell the abuser how harmful his actions were and how the trauma can affect the child, the adolescent, the adult. She wrote this letter.

Shirley's letter

Dear Abuser,

For many years I have hated you, and for many years I wanted to march in on you when your shop was full of people and vent all my hatred upon you, to humiliate you as you humiliated me. I wanted to scream out the hurt you caused and show you that we, the children of abuse, grow up but we don't ever forget.

Have you any idea of the damage you have done? Did you really think it was such a harmless bit of fun to grope round a small child's body? Did you really think that you could do that leaving a child's mind and soul untouched? If there is any shred of human decency left in you, and if you truly understood the damage you inflicted, you would never do such a thing again. So, I am going to tell you about the damage you have done to me.

You polluted my mind with things I knew nothing about, things no child should have to know. In violating me you caused me to feel ashamed and dirty, and that sense of feeling unclean never diminished. I grew up both rejecting my body and yet desperately trying to control it. One of the greatest crimes you committed was that you caused me to doubt my self-worth. It was not I who was degraded, whose worth as a person was diminished. Now I can hold my head up knowing I did nothing wrong.

I felt guilty. You knew that children are told never to take sweets from strangers, so you gave me a sweet after abusing me knowing I wouldn't refuse it. Knowing that in taking it I would be doing something I knew to be wrong, thus ensuring my silence and my guilt. Was that all I was worth to you, a penny chew? In giving me that sweet you put me in the wrong so I could never tell what you had done.

Are you so sure it has all been worth it? For a few minutes of sexual excitement, for a moment of power over a child, you inflicted so much harm, damaged my life and the lives of so many others. You will not be able to lay the blame on the child all your life. We, the abused, refuse to accept all the hurt, anguish and guilt you have tried to force upon us. We, the abused, can heal, we can find peace, we can be free; while you, the abuser, can never rest. You must always hide from yourself, from your guilt, from your shame; for if you knew their true measure they would surely overwhelm you.

I am on my way to freedom. Freedom from you, from all the pain, guilt, hatred and fear you inspired. I am free now to love a man without fearing him. Shirley

Luke felt angry about how the abuse had made him hate himself and question his sexuality. Writing this letter helped Luke vent his anger and place the responsibility for the abuse back on to his abuser.

Luke's letter

I've needed to talk to you for a while now. You're probably wondering what about or maybe you know.

Do you remember the pub, 'The Red Lion', where we used to live? That's where it all started. That's where you started touching my penis, masturbating me, trying to kiss me, telling your perverted stories, walking through the flat with virtually nothing on, always looking for an opportunity. I know it didn't just happen to me.

Can you remember how old I was? No, you probably can't. Your only reason for doing it was your own sexual gratification. You didn't even think about how it might affect me. I bet it never crossed your mind what you were really doing – fucking up my life, condemning me to wonder about my own sexuality. You left me stranded. I'd never thought about sex until *you* started abusing me and then all I knew was what you taught me – how to blame myself. Every day I woke up hating myself for what I'd done. I enjoyed what you did and I hate myself for that. I hate myself for something *you* did. If you think back, you'll remember I was only 11 years old and ever since I've taken responsibility for something you did. I'll never blame another child the way I've blamed myself, the way I still blame myself. So, for the past 15 years I've put the whole experience down to me being homosexual but that's wrong, I'm not. You sexually abused me. You were to blame.

I want you to know that I'm not keeping this secret any more. I've been living in a hell that you started because you couldn't control your own sexual urges, but you could control a lonely 11-year-old boy. You're a bastard and I hate you. There's a big difference now. You're going to be the scared one. Now it's your turn to worry about the future. The crime you committed is a crime worse than any other. To kill someone is to take away their life, that's straightforward by comparison. To abuse a child, you don't give them the release of death, you send them to death on earth. What really upsets me is I know that I can't hurt you the way I want to. I can't make you feel this pain. Luke

Katarina wanted to tell her abuser, her brother, how he had damaged her life. She wanted to express her anger and her sadness at being unable to relate to him as a brother.

Katarina's letter

Brother,
I was asked to write to you and, thinking about it, I agree that it is a good thing to tell you what I think about you and what damage you have done to me.

You have been so clever; not only abusing my body but also making sure I would grow up with fear in my heart and no self-esteem. For 20 years after the abuse I still thought of myself as less worthy than other people. You made sure that if you were around I felt like a worm about to be stepped on. I wanted to see you dead, but my fear of you made it impossible to attack you in any other way than in my mind. I was still helpless.

If only you had shown some form of remorse, treated me with kindness when we were grown up. Although I hated you there was a part in me that desperately wanted to forgive you, to be liked by you, to make a new start and become at last a brother and sister in the way I had seen in other families. Yet I know if I had told you what damage your abuse did to me you would have done no more than shrug your shoulders and say 'So what?'
Katarina

In her letter, Katarina went on to describe in detail how his abuse had affected her whole life and expressed her anger to him for this. Having talked about her abuse and worked through her feelings, Katarina's feelings towards her brother have changed:

Of course I am still angry. But it is not the same kind of anger any more that I used to feel. The kind of anger I feel now is anger at someone who has done me wrong, who knew it full well and did not care. It is the healthy kind of anger not the kind that sees no reason and is nothing but blind fury. If I see him in the street, when I go back to my hometown, I am now strong enough to look him in the eyes. **Katarina**

Regaining your power from the abuser

Some survivors have no contact with their abusers, or their abusers are now dead. Others may see their abusers occasionally or on a regular basis, especially if the abuser is a family member or lives locally. Thinking about the abuser, whether he or she is alive or dead, can make survivors feel frightened, vulnerable or angry. Even survivors who feel very angry can quickly regress to feeling child-like, powerless and frightened when they actually see their abuser, as Anthony discovered. Some survivors continue to see or hear their abusers even though the abuser is dead, and these hallucinations can be terrifying and paralysing. (See Chapter 8, 'Anxiety, fears and trauma', for information and advice on coping with hallucinations.)

The exercise below aims to help you overcome feelings of fear towards your abuser and to feel more empowered. It also helps to reinforce the knowledge that what happened to you was not right and that you were not to blame for being abused. Sexual abuse is a crime, the perpetrator has committed illegal acts.

It is important that the exercise below is done on paper or in your imagination, not in person with your abuser. This means *you* are in control of what happens. Confronting your abuser in imagination can be a very powerful and liberating experience for survivors. Confronting your abuser in person is a very different matter and can be dangerous for you, both physically and psychologically. The exercise is not aimed at helping you to confront your abuser in person but at helping you feel more powerful by understanding and expressing your thoughts and feelings about the abuse and the abuser.

Exercise: Standing up to your abuser in imagination

1 *What do you want to say?*
   Think carefully about exactly what you want to say to your abuser. Do you want to express how you feel about the abuse?

Do you want to tell the abuser how he or she has damaged your life? Write down exactly what you want to say as a series of short statements – for example, 'You raped me. I have a lot of problems because of what you did to me. You are responsible.'

2 *The abuser's response*

When abusers are confronted about the abuse in person they rarely admit to what they have done. They usually deny that the abuse ever happened or minimize what really happened by pretending it wasn't sexual abuse but something innocent or loving. Some abusers blame the survivor for what happened, often by suggesting the survivor wanted the abuse or caused it to happen in some way – these may be the same things the abuser said to the survivor as a child. Some abusers threaten the survivor for speaking out about the abuse and, again, this may be a familiar pattern, experienced from childhood. Think about how your abuser might respond if he or she were challenged and write this down.

3 *Your assertive replies*

Think about how you could reply assertively and write down your replies. Learning how to challenge abusers' reactions by responding assertively (in the exercise, not in person) can help you feel more in control and more powerful in relation to your abuser. Keep your replies simple. Deny what isn't true, and state what is true. Do not be side-tracked or think you have to justify how you feel.

Here are some examples of steps 2 and 3.

Abuser's reactions	**Possible assertive replies**
Denying	
'I did not touch you.'	'Yes, you did. You had intercourse with me.'
'I don't know what you're talking about.'	'Yes, you do. You made me touch your penis.'
'You are a liar/mentally ill/ imagining it.'	'I am not a liar/mentally ill/ imagining it, you did touch my private parts.'
'You are suffering from false memory syndrome.'	'No I am not. You raped me.'

Abuser's reactions	Possible assertive replies
Minimizing	
'I was only tickling you.'	'You did not only tickle me. You rubbed my genitals.'
'I was teaching you the facts of life.'	'You were not teaching me the facts of life. You sexually abused me.'
'I was only playing with you.'	'You were not only playing with me. You masturbated over me.'
Blaming	
'You enjoyed it.'	'You were responsible. You sexually abused me.'
'You kept taking your clothes off in front of me. You asked for it.'	'You were an adult and you sexually abused a child.'
Threatening	
'No one will speak to you again.'	'I am not to blame. You are responsible for the abuse.'
'I'll tell your parents what you've done.'	'You are responsible for the abuse. You are to blame.'

4 *Role-play confrontation*
After you have done this, try role-playing the confrontation with a friend. Get a friend to pretend to be the abuser and act out the confrontation. Practise all the abuser's possible reactions, however unlikely or upsetting they are, and how you would respond. You may find this is more difficult than you think. Although this is an imaginary confrontation, you may experience all the feelings of fear and vulnerability that you felt as a child. Keep practising. As you feel more able to stand up to your abuser in imagination, you will begin to let go of your fear and feel more powerful.

Confronting the abuser in person

Some survivors feel they need to confront their abusers in person. This is not a necessary part of the healing process and can be very damaging to the survivor if it is done at the wrong time, with unrealistic expectations or without the right preparation. Some perpetrators may be violent.

Survivors' expectations of what might happen can be very wrong. They often think that the abuser will be hurt and upset if they confront him or her, and assume the abuser must feel dreadful about what he or she has done. As we have seen, though, abusers usually deny what they have done however strong the evidence against them. If the abuser does admit to the abuse at all, he or she will probably minimize it. The abuser might also try to blame or threaten you. These reactions could be devastating if you are not prepared for them or if you still feel guilty, unsure about your memories and feelings, or intimidated by the abuser.

We advise against confronting your abuser in person, but if you decide that you want to do this, IT IS VERY IMPORTANT THAT YOU DO NOT DO THIS UNTIL YOU ARE FULLY PREPARED. In this section, we will look at why some survivors want to confront their abusers, how to prepare to confront your abuser and what happened when some of the Wakefield survivors took action.

WHY CONFRONT THE ABUSER?
Pam remembers how she talked to friends at work about her plans to confront her abuser.

> One of my colleagues said 'You only want to confront your father to split him and your mother up, to teach him a lesson.' I replied, nearly in tears, 'No, that isn't the reason I want to confront him. I want to get over the anxieties I have about men in general, I look at men that I don't know and think of them as potential child abusers.' **Pam**

Like Pam, some survivors want to confront their abusers to overcome their fear of that person and of people in general. Some survivors decide to confront their abusers to protect other children, especially when they know that he or she has already abused many victims.

> I knew my father had abused a lot of other members of my family and I suspected he was still doing so. I could protect my own children from him but how could I protect everyone else? I asked my sister to come with me to support me when I confronted him.

> Our aim was not to hurt him but to stop him hurting anyone else.
> He did admit he had done some things to his daughters which he
> regretted, but denied abusing anyone else. He said the others just
> wanted to make trouble and were out to get him. We told him we
> were watching him and that I was not going to keep quiet if he
> continued abusing. **Kate**

There were other benefits for Kate from this confrontation:

> I did not say all the things I wanted to say but I was quite sur-
> prised to find that I had passed the burden of guilt back to him,
> where it rightly belongs. I felt strong. The power relationship
> between us changed after this. He seemed to avoid me, rather
> than me having to avoid him. **Kate**

Sexual abuse occurs in secret. The abuser gets the child to comply
by using some form of power (adult authority, manipulation,
physical strength, threats), leaving the victim feeling powerless and
controlled by the abuser. Often the victims feel they are under the
abuser's power for the rest of their lives. Confronting the abuser
can break the secret *and* take this power away from him or her.
Although Kate had primarily gone to confront her abuser to protect
other children and young people, she also found the power relationship between her and her father had reversed.

Exercise: Why do you want to confront your abuser?

1 Write down what you are aiming to achieve by confronting your
   abuser.
2 For each aim, ask yourself, 'Is this realistic?' For example, if you
   want the abuser to say sorry, this isn't very realistic as he or she
   is highly unlikely to do so.
3 Ask yourself if there is any better or easier way to achieve
   your aim. For example, it might be better to contact the local
   authority child protection unit, the NSPCC or the police in order
   to protect other children and young people (see 'Sources of help'
   at the back of this book). You may be able to deal with your
   anger as effectively by standing up to your abuser in imagination, as described earlier.

Common reasons survivors give for wanting to confront abusers
include:

- to break the silence and, with it, the hold the abuser may still have over them;
- to reverse the power relationship;
- to rid themselves of the fear they still have inside – the fear an abused child has of his or her adult abuser;
- to protect other children and young people from the abuser;
- to help them get over their own fears and anxieties about people in general;
- to express their own anger and distress;
- to get the abuser to acknowledge what he or she has done and to see the harm he or she has caused;
- to clear the air and help resolve their feelings towards the abuser.

Some of these aims are unlikely to be achieved. Abusers will rarely admit to the abuse, so survivors must be prepared for all possible reactions. Survivors are very likely be disappointed if they hope the abuser will acknowledge the harm he or she has done. Make sure your aims are realistic and you have explored the alternatives before you decide to go ahead with the confrontation.

Preparing for a confrontation

We do not recommend that you literally confront your abuser, but if you are determined to do so, please make sure you are fully prepared and that you are not placing yourself in any danger. You will need to pay attention to the points below.

YOUR OWN FEELINGS

It is important that you do not plan to confront your abuser until you have worked through your own feelings about the abuse. It would be best to have some counselling first, or to at least have read this book and talked to others about the abuse. You need to feel certain that the abuse was not your fault and that the abuser was responsible for what happened. The abuser may accuse you of being a liar, say you are crazy or blame you for the abuse. You will end up feeling much worse if you are in any doubt about what happened and who was responsible.

It is also important that you do not see the abuser if you are full of rage. The purpose is to talk to him or her, not to physically attack them. Attacking the abuser could put you in physical danger and have legal consequences. It will also leave you feeling helpless and out of control again. Make sure you have first worked through the exercises in this chapter on expressing your feelings (talking to a cushion and writing letters).

SUPPORT

If you know of anyone else who has been abused by the same person, ask them to confront the abuser with you. Go through all the preparations with them. If you have a partner or friend with you when you confront the abuser, make sure they understand they are there for support only. It will not help you feel empowered if another person takes over and confronts the abuser or deals with the abuser's reactions. If you are going to confront the abuser alone, have someone you trust in the next room. Afterwards you will need someone to talk to about how you feel, so make sure there will be someone available to support you.

PRACTISE

Be clear about what you want to say to your abuser and be prepared for whatever response he or she might give. Use the exercise on standing up to your abuser in imagination to prepare yourself, and practise again and again with a friend or therapist by role-playing the confrontation. Do not go ahead with the confrontation until you feel certain that you can handle whatever the abuser might say.

A few abusers break down, cry and say they are sorry when they are confronted. Survivors may then feel pity for the abusers and regret hurting them. It is the abuser who hurt you; if he or she is upset, it is because of what he or she has done. Remember that abusers manipulate their victims so they can sexually abuse them. Abusers may cry because they are genuinely sorry or they may cry to manipulate their victims into feeling sorry for them and therefore retract what they have said. Abusers may also cry for themselves because they are frightened of other people knowing what they have done or are terrified of being prosecuted by the police. You could respond by saying, for example:

- 'You are upset because of what *you* have done.'

- 'Don't expect me to comfort you, *you* abused me.'
- 'Well, you should be upset about this.'

PLAN

Plan in detail where, when and how you are going to confront the abuser. Choose a place where you feel comfortable and safe, your home or neutral territory. Some survivors choose to confront their abusers in a public place with a friend nearby for added protection.

VERY IMPORTANT: Do not confront someone who may be violent.

PAM'S CONFRONTATION

Pam rang her parents and told them to come round to see her that evening at 8.30 p.m.

> We hadn't had contact for over two years. My immediate thought was – would I break down?
>
> I set my husband on making coffee to keep him out of the way – I had to do this alone. My mother sat beside my father in the lounge so I dismissed her immediately to the dining room. I then confronted my father with exactly what he'd done to me. He'd raped me and sucked my body. I told him how this had affected me, particularly over the past two years when I had had a nervous breakdown. I told him that I became agoraphobic and I couldn't have a sexual relationship with my husband because all I saw was my father's face. I told him I hated him so much.
>
> He sat there for approximately an hour and listened to me. I then told him I wanted to tell my mother in front of him to prove to her I wasn't lying. I'd actually told her about it at the time it first happened and many times since, but she'd dismissed me as a liar.
>
> My father more or less made his admission of guilt by non-denial. But I was pleased, because normally you can't talk to him without him blowing his top. He was completely devastated and I thought, 'Well, now you can walk round with it on your conscience for the rest of your life.' I told them both they were lucky to be alive walking out of my house, because all I wanted to do was kick their teeth in or stab them both to death. I hated them so much. Their reaction was that they didn't blame me. **Pam**

Pam's father did not admit his guilt but neither did he deny it. Pam had at last managed to express her anger and distress to her parents, and this marked a turning point in her relationship with them and in her own feelings.

> When they had gone, I felt like I'd been carrying a massive rucksack and somebody had just taken it off me. I felt absolutely marvellous. I felt I'd really achieved something. All I ever wanted was a mum and dad who cared and loved me. Up to the present the change in them is unbelievable, but for the better, and I feel a lot better within myself. There is life after abuse and this is what it took for me to find that out. **Pam**

Pam's husband, Brian, describes the change in her relationship with her parents after the confrontation.

> The big turning point came when Pam decided to confront the abuser, her father. She got 24 years of anger off her chest in as many minutes. Now she is a changed woman, never to be intimidated by her parents again. In fact, they are now a bit unnerved by her and at her beck and call. Since then there has been some form of family relationship. On my part it is toleration because they are Pam's parents. On her part – they are always her parents in the end. **Brian**

CLAIRE AND JOAN'S CONFRONTATION

Sisters Claire and Joan were both sexually abused as children by their brother-in-law Tony, the husband of their eldest sister. They decided to confront Tony in person because Joan was still feeling depressed and powerless at the end of her group therapy, and because they were worried he might be abusing his own children. As Claire said:

> I want to confront him, to show him how bad it is and to stop him if he's still doing it. I don't want him to think he has escaped. I want him to feel ashamed of what he did. **Claire**

Several meetings were held to discuss their expectations about what might happen, and to brief their husbands. The meetings were also to plan what they wanted to say and to practise assertive ways of dealing with all of Tony's possible reactions. Claire and Joan initially thought Tony would admit what he had done and get upset. Without the meetings and practice, they would not have been prepared for what did happen.

My younger sister Joan and I were to confront our abuser, Tony, together. We were quite scared but we felt ready to go ahead with it. We both felt we needed to do this and in a strange way I was looking forward to it. The scene was set at Joan's house. Her husband had left the house, but while we waited for Tony to arrive we were wishing that her husband had stayed. Later we were very proud of ourselves for doing it alone. As we saw Tony walk down the garden path Joan decided to calm herself down by doing a few of the breathing exercises we had learned at group therapy.

Tony had no idea why we wanted to see him but we wasted no time. I was the first to speak and I told him that Joan and I were seeing a psychologist because of what he had done to us as children. Colour drained from his face and I felt stronger. He said, quite annoyed, that he didn't know what we were talking about and that he'd never done anything to us. Joan had to spell it out and all the time he was denying it. He said he was only tickling us. By this time, he was standing at the door and saying he was leaving. Joan suddenly became very strong and confident and continued to tell him how well we remembered where and when those awful things took place and he got very frightened and raised his voice.

He continued to trip himself up with his lies and as he kept changing his story, he seemed to get smaller and smaller, weaker and weaker. We felt more sure of his guilt than ever now. We kept saying over again 'Yes, you did it'. He said we were both insane and he felt sorry for us. Then he used his last weapon when he said, 'I'll tell your mum and dad – what will they say about what you've done?'

Something clicked inside me – I had heard this before from him, all those years ago. Except this time, instead of feeling guilty, I felt more sure I was doing the right thing and said 'Yes, what would they say to you, if they knew what *you* did to their children?'

We continued to surprise him by telling him we knew of two other women who had been his victims. We told him we could take him to court and that we were worried about his own daughters. He still denied everything and said he was going to get his wife, Rita (our sister). She arrived shortly, alone. He had told her what had been said and swore blind to her that he hadn't done anything.

When it was all over I felt sorry for my sister Rita. I wanted to put my arms around her but I couldn't, because she still didn't say she believed us. I still felt we had done the right thing.

It was a big relief to know it was all over and I wouldn't have to do it again. I was full of confidence and thought we performed well. We couldn't have done it any better and we did it alone, without our men behind us. Now Tony knows how much he hurt us and spoiled Joan's life and now he's spoiled his own. It feels really great to put the guilt on to him. It's changed my life.

I don't blush very much these days. Each day I get a little more confident and like myself better. I released a lot of anger on that day and now I feel much calmer. It's changing Joan's life too. The very next day she went swimming and instead of rushing into the water, so that no one could see her body, she idled about for a while and could look at people in the water and hold her head up high. She didn't feel ashamed any more.

I don't feel like keeping it a secret any more. In fact, I want to tell all the family except Mum and Dad – not because of shame this time but to protect them from feeling they let us down by failing to protect us from this pathetic person. **Claire**

Their sister, Rita, soon believed them, and Claire and Joan made sure Tony's own children were safe by contacting social services (Chapter 16, 'Working towards prevention', describes the procedures for protecting children).

During the confrontation, Tony seemed to the sisters to become smaller and weaker, while they felt themselves growing bigger and stronger. Claire and Joan had anticipated all of Tony's possible responses and practised how they would reply, so it did not matter that he denied abusing them. What was important was that they were able to confront him and show him and themselves that they were no longer ashamed and were not responsible for the abuse. Joan got her power back and immediately began improving. Her depression lifted and she began to feel more confident every day.

JOANNE'S ATTEMPTED PROSECUTION

Joanne had spent her childhood in fear of her stepfather, Ken, who was physically violent as well as sexually abusive. As an adult, she had told her mother and family what had happened to her but was then shunned by them and still felt she carried the blame for the abuse.

Joanne decided not to confront her stepfather directly as he was a violent man. However, she still wanted Ken and her family to acknowledge that it was Ken, and not she, who was responsible for the abuse, so she went to the police and gave a statement. Unfortunately, the case was never brought to court because of lack of supporting evidence. Joanne, however, was not disheartened by this because Ken had been arrested and her accusation made public. She expressed her feelings by writing a letter without sending it.

Joanne's letter

Dear Ken,
Well, no doubt you are feeling very relieved at the moment, after hearing that you're not going to be prosecuted after all, even though you sexually abused me for years. At the beginning of the survivors' group I would have been devastated if I'd known that the case wouldn't go to court but now, much to my surprise, I don't feel bitter. I feel I've made my point to you. You now know how much I hate you and that, if possible, I would have seen you imprisoned once again. I felt a great deal of satisfaction when I heard that you'd had to have minor surgery through stomach pains due to the 'stress and worry' you've been going through for the past 10 months. This gave me pleasure to hear; at least you've suffered in some way after all the suffering you caused me and all those around you.

For all those years, I was absolutely terrified of you. Well now I feel so proud and full of strength to have stood up to you. For the past year, I've been the one who has had power over you. My actions have brought worry and fear to you. For years, you told me that if I spoke about it 'no one would ever want to have anything to do with me ever again'. How it delights me when I know you now realize that I can discuss this terrible 'secret' with others and with members of our family. How false those threats were but as a child these and other threats seemed very real. It hurts to realize how commonly these threats are made by you and your fellow abusers.

I thank my lucky stars daily that I've received help. I'm relieved to say that I sincerely feel as if I've been 're-born' at the age of 31. At least you haven't ruined the whole of my life. I'll never forgive you for what you've done to me and the way you've blighted my life up until now with my husband and my own children. They have seen me during my periods of depression and sadness, though not any more. You can't hurt *me* any more. I'm finally rid of you. I don't feel I'll ever be able to forgive you, but

I'm certainly on the way to forgetting about what you did and the problems you have caused. I am now getting on with my life and, perhaps more importantly, I'm aware that my life is now more rich than yours. Joanne

Joanne had anticipated all the things that could happen if she gave a statement to the police, so that even though the case was dropped before it got to court, confronting her abuser in this way helped Joanne regain her own power. After the police had interviewed Ken, Joanne wrote:

He now knows he doesn't have a hold over me any more. He can no longer frighten me with the threat that everyone will blame me and reject me if I tell about the abuse.

Summary

Abusers do not fit a stereotype. They can be men and women of any age, class, race or religion. They can have many different personality characteristics and lifestyles. The feelings survivors have towards their abusers can be just as varied. They may have a conflicting mixture of feelings including hate, love, fear, guilt, concern, disgust, betrayal, pity and anger. The exercises suggested in this chapter can help survivors to explore and understand their feelings towards their abusers; to express their feelings and so release some of their pain; and to regain their personal power.

Suggestions

- Explore your feelings towards your abuser using the exercises described in this chapter (talking to a cushion or writing a letter to the abuser) or by talking to a counsellor or therapist.
- To help you regain your power from your abuser, try the exercise on standing up to your abuser in imagination.
- We do not recommend that you confront your abuser face to face. If, however, you have decided to do this, please be very careful and follow the guidelines in the chapter. DO NOT confront your abuser without full preparation – it will only cause you more emotional distress. DO NOT confront an abuser who is likely to be violent.

- There are exercises in the chapter on 'Abusers' in the *Breaking Free Workbook* that take you step by step through the suggestions above.

- If you are feeling powerless or out of control, or you are having hallucinations of the abuser, EMDR therapy can be very helpful in reducing the power of your emotions, eliminating the hallucinations and allowing you to feel in control again. Read the 'Getting help' section of the next chapter, 'Overcoming the problems'. (Chapter 8 also has more information on coping with hallucinations.)

- If you know or suspect that your abuser is currently abusing another child, protect the child by informing your local authority child protection team or the NSPCC or get some advice by contacting one of the telephone helplines listed in the 'Sources of help' section at the back of the book. Chapter 16, 'Working towards prevention', contains more information on protecting children and young people.

Part 5
BREAKING FREE

15

Overcoming the problems

> Before I went for therapy I thought I would never feel strong
> enough to take charge of my own life. I wouldn't have believed it
> was possible for my life to change so much. **Jane**

You *can* learn to feel better about yourself and overcome the problems resulting from the sexual abuse. In this chapter, we look at
how survivors have broken free from their problems and regained
their own power. We discuss how you could find a psychotherapist
if you feel ready to take that step now.

Survivors describe what it was about being in a therapy group
that helped them, and how they have changed after individual
or group therapy. Some of the quotations and information in this
chapter derive from research conducted on the Wakefield survivor
groups by clinical psychologist Sally Pinnell.

Getting help

We have seen how childhood sexual abuse results in adult survivors feeling bad about themselves and experiencing problems in
many areas of their lives. Some survivors are only mildly affected
by the abuse, but others hate themselves and feel that their lives
have been destroyed by the abuse. How can you begin to break free
from the impact of the sexual abuse and take back control of your
life? Reading this book and working through the exercises is a start.
Talking to a trusted friend or family member may also help, by
breaking the secret and allowing you to feel accepted by someone
who knows what has happened to you.

For some survivors, this may be enough, but others will need
to get further help by seeking individual therapy or joining a survivors' group. Before you decide you do not need any further help,
talk it over (in person or on a telephone helpline) with someone
who could offer help. You may find it difficult to go for help

because you feel ashamed and worthless or think your problems are insignificant.

> I was afraid I would be wasting the psychologist's time. I was not worthy of nice people wasting their valuable time on a disgusting person like me. **Eileen**

Feeling unworthy is one of the consequences of being sexually abused. You do deserve help.

> If you are being abused in any way or have been abused, no matter how long ago it happened, please tell someone and get some help. You owe it to yourself. **Joan**

FINDING A THERAPIST

We hope that reading this book has encouraged you to take the next step and find a therapist to help you put the abuse and its consequences behind you. You deserve it! If the person you choose to speak to does not believe you, or responds inappropriately, find another person and keep on telling until someone listens and supports you. If you begin therapy and find the therapist, or type of therapy, is unhelpful, discuss this with them or find another therapist. If you have any concerns about the therapist's behaviour, discuss this with a friend or with a professional (for example, your doctor). It is very important that you check a therapist is qualified and accredited by a professional body.

Registration/accreditation

Being registered/accredited with a professional body means an individual must have achieved a substantial level of training and experience approved by their member organization. All the professional organizations hold a list of approved therapists – you can check their websites to find a therapist in your area. The websites for the main professional bodies for counselling and psychotherapy are listed in the 'Sources of help' section at the back of the book, together with other agencies that provide therapy.

You can find a therapist via your GP; this could be a referral to a clinical psychologist, a counsellor, a cognitive behavioural therapist, a psychotherapist, a mental health worker, or IAPT (Improving Access to Psychological Therapy) services. In some areas, you can self-refer to IAPT services. Your GP may refer you to a therapist in the National Health Service (NHS; all NHS therapists are qualified and accredited), or provide you with a list of private therapists (whose qualifications and accreditation you may need to check). You may be able to find a therapist at low or no cost via a local charity or voluntary agency; or you may have the funds to pay for a private therapist yourself. Do not be afraid to ask to see a woman if you feel uncomfortable talking to a man (or vice versa).

There are a wide range of therapies that can help with many of the consequences of child sexual abuse, including relationship issues. What is important is finding the form of therapy that suits you and a therapist you can learn to feel comfortable with, and ensuring the therapist is qualified and accredited. Many of the suggestions and exercises in this book are based on a CBT approach. Psychodynamic or humanistic therapies, like Gestalt or transactional analysis, might help with the impact of abuse on relationships and some of the more complex issues that develop in those who have experienced long-term abuse or abuse within the family.

GETTING HELP WITH TRAUMA OR PTSD SYMPTOMS
The exercises in this book can help with trauma and PTSD symptoms but it can take a long time to resolve these symptoms if the experiences are 'stuck' in the information-processing system of the brain. Specialist help is recommended to reduce the symptoms of trauma. If you are struggling with PTSD or symptoms of trauma such as flashbacks, nightmares or intrusive images (see Box 2 in Chapter 2), you will benefit from some therapy specifically focused on the effects of trauma. The only therapies recommended in National Institute for Health and Care Excellence (NICE) guidelines (<www.nice.org.uk/guidance>) for PTSD are EMDR therapy (see below) and trauma-focused CBT. Your GP may be able to refer you for EMDR or trauma-focused CBT; otherwise find an accredited CBT therapist or an accredited EMDR therapist.

EMDR therapy

EMDR therapy is a powerful psychological treatment that was developed in the 1980s by the American psychologist Dr Francine Shapiro. You do not have to talk in any detail about the abuse, and during the treatment itself there is very little talking involved. It is very effective in resolving the problems resulting from child abuse or any other traumas.

Chapter 2 describes how certain functions of the brain are disrupted when a person experiences a trauma. This results in the experience not being processed and filed away properly. EMDR utilizes the body's natural healing ability and allows the brain to heal the effects of trauma effectively and rapidly. It works directly with the brain and nervous system to allow the inherent adaptive information-processing system to complete the processing of the trauma so the incident quickly becomes 'just a memory' and can be remembered without the accompanying distress.

How EMDR works

EMDR is a complex and powerful process (and therefore should only be conducted by therapists who have completed an accredited training course). The essence of the approach is to stimulate the information-processing system in the brain (this is non-intrusive and painless!) and, at the same time, inform the brain about the target event you wish to process and lay down as a memory.

Technique – alternate bilateral stimulation

The technique used to enable the brain to go into information-processing mode and repair any brain disruption caused by trauma or difficult experiences is called alternate bilateral stimulation. The brain is in two halves, connected by a thick band of nerve fibres called the corpus callosum, and bilateral stimulation consists of sending a signal via the senses to each side of the brain in turn. When she developed EMDR therapy, Francine Shapiro used eye movements (hence the name) to stimulate one side of the brain after the other, but sounds or tactile stimulation (using tapping) may also be used. Whichever sense is used to input into the brain, the purpose is to stimulate one side of the brain after the other. The bilateral stimulation activates the blocked information-processing system so it can complete the job of processing the memory of the trauma by encouraging communication between the two halves of the brain via the connecting band of nerve fibres.

Before the bilateral stimulation is started, we need to let the brain know what information we want to process. To do this, we activate the neural networks (patterns of brain cells) relating to the traumatic event by choosing a target. When the 'target' or situation to be processed has been selected (for example, the first time the person was abused), the neural networks representing the event are activated by identifying the image that represents the event, the negative beliefs that go with it, the related emotions and any bodily sensations. The bilateral stimulation then facilitates the brain in rapidly completing the disrupted processing, and the traumatic event can be laid down as an old memory without the accompanying distress. When EMDR on this target is completed, the person can usually recall or discuss the target event in a more dispassionate manner and with the knowledge the event is now over.

EMDR UK and Ireland (at: <www.emdrassociation.org.uk>) can help you find an accredited EMDR therapist in your area (see the 'Sources of help' section at the back of the book for how to find EMDR therapists in Europe, the USA and other non-European countries).

HOW CAN ANYTHING HELP?

I couldn't believe that just talking would help, it did, it does. I like myself, I did nothing wrong. **Jocelyn**

If you were sexually abused as a child, nothing can change that fact. What can change is the way you see yourself, the way you understand what happened during the abuse, and the way you feel about yourself and others. Building up a relationship with someone who knows your background and problems (rather than someone who just knows the 'front' that many survivors hide behind) can help you overcome problems in trusting others.

Understanding, as an adult, the events of your childhood will help you see that you were not to blame for the abuse, you were not responsible; and in time the feelings of guilt, shame and self-blame will also change. You can conquer problems relating to your sexuality and your sexual behaviour by working on your feelings about yourself. Your feelings of powerlessness will fade as you learn to face up to your fears, rather than avoiding them, and as you begin to take control of your own life, your own problems and your own emotions. Your own power will grow as you assert yourself in the world and discover who you really are without the burden of shame and fear. Reading this book, going for therapy or joining a group *can* help you overcome your problems.

WRITING

> Writing is the thing I've found really helpful, once I started writing I couldn't stop. It really surprised me – I could write better than I could talk. **Claire**

Writing can help you overcome your problems, whether you are working on these alone or with the help of others. You do not need to write by hand – you can always type into a personal file on your computer, phone or tablet. Survivors have found writing especially helpful in allowing them to remember their experiences, explore and express their feelings, face up to their fears, and accept their experiences and themselves. In Chapter 1, we suggested you do the written exercises at the end of each chapter. This can be difficult for some people, but many survivors find this an important part of the healing process. Some survivors are too frightened of writing their thoughts down. They are frightened that someone else will see them, or are afraid that if their thoughts are written down they will have to face up to the fact that the events really happened.

> I found writing terrifying. I would scrawl things down but I couldn't look at them or else I would throw them away. **Colleen**

Many survivors feel the need to throw away or destroy their writings at first. You could keep a stamped addressed envelope ready and post them to someone you trust (a therapist if you have one) as soon as you've written them, or email them to a trusted person if you feel the need to delete the file on your computer. You can ask the person who receives the writing to read them, or just hold on to them until you are ready to read them again or show them to someone else.

> I always used to burn my writings but then I started posting them to my therapist as soon as I'd written them. Posting them still felt like I was getting rid of them again but then they arrived at her office and it was there in black and white – not hidden any more. It was still my secret when I burnt them so I was pleased when I could let my therapist read them. I felt so much better that it wasn't hidden. Everything before had to be a secret – no openness at all. **Lucy**

You may find it difficult to begin writing. It's difficult to get started, you're thinking about who is going to see it, but once you start you don't know where to stop. One of the girls from an earlier group has kept all her writings and says she can see how much she has improved. One girl says she writes down her thoughts when her mind is racing and it helps her to stop thinking about it. I'm going to try that at the times when I can't concentrate. **Claire**

Writing becomes a way of helping you cope with your thoughts and feelings and a way of releasing all the secret fears and memories.

At first I tended not to think about things so they wouldn't hurt as much. Now I think things out and write them down, not push them down. It's best to deal with things. I'm quite good at that now. **Claire**

Writing can help survivors to remember more about their child-hoods and to see the past in a new light.

So I started writing. It was really helpful. I could go back and remember. Once I started writing I couldn't stop. It wasn't just about the abuse it was about all my childhood. By writing it down I really could see why it wasn't my fault – why it happened and why I couldn't tell. That was the best part, it was a real help. **Mavis**

If you have not been able to do the written exercises at the end of the chapters, why not try again now? It may suit some of you to just read through this book and then try all the exercises later on. You may also want to try the exercises in the *Breaking Free Workbook*, which are more detailed and lead you step by step through a process of tackling and overcoming your difficulties. If you find writing dif-ficult, look at the alternatives to writing described in Chapter 1.

Joining a survivors' group

After I saw my therapist three or four times, she suggested I joined a group but I didn't want to go. The idea of being in a group of other women really frightened me. But I eventually said 'Yes' and it was the best thing I've ever done. **Jocelyn**

Not everyone would like to join a group or has the opportunity to join one. We have found that survivors benefit a great deal from being in a group and overcome their problems much more quickly.

FEARS ABOUT JOINING A GROUP

> I saw my therapist four times before I joined the group. I was terrified of being in a group. I didn't want to speak to anyone else about it. It was this secret between the psychologist and me and nobody else.
>
> I was frightened of the group and didn't think it would help but I would have given anything a go as I'd got so desperate. I don't know what I expected. I was so afraid of anyone knowing what had happened to me. I was so ashamed of it. It was my secret. What would they think of me? I thought they would blame me for letting it happen. **Lucy**

Many people are nervous or extremely frightened at the thought of joining a group. Sexual abuse occurs in secret, and the feelings of shame arise partly from keeping this secret. Widening the circle of people who know about the secret by joining a group can be very frightening, but feeling accepted by other people who know the secret can help reduce the feeling of shame.

> I didn't want to go to the group at first because it was increasing the number of people who knew what had happened to me. My psychologist said she could sit there and talk to me about how other survivors feel but it would be different for me to talk to the women myself, to actually go into a room with other survivors, who know I have been abused too and have the same feelings.
>
> I didn't know if I would get to the first group meeting until I actually got there. Walking into the room I realized everyone was in the same boat. I didn't feel threatened when I walked in but I didn't enjoy it. I felt I'd come this far and had to do it. **Jocelyn**

Survivors often fear that someone else in the group will know them or talk about them outside the group.

> I am a professional woman and I had fears of joining a group in case someone from the group recognized me in the street and discussed me in public. Everyone would know what *I* had done. The group discussed confidentiality and the therapists asked every member present to respect each other. They said it was unlikely that anyone would discuss another group member in public as they had all suffered the same or similar experiences. This was very reassuring to me and put me at ease immediately. **Eileen**

Many people say they should not be part of a survivors' group because they feel a fraud. They think they shouldn't be in the group because they can't remember what happened during their abuse, or they think their abuse was not as serious as everyone else's.

> The first week at the group I knew I had been abused but with not remembering much about it I didn't know if it had *really* happened and that was my big fear. At first you feel everyone else is much worse than you and then you get it into perspective and realize that whatever the form of the abuse it has affected each of us. **Jocelyn**

Many survivors feel that they are different from everyone else or that their abuse was different. In the group, survivors become aware that they have many feelings in common and that whatever has happened to each of them, it was just another form of sexual abuse.

It may help you overcome your fears about joining a group if you can arrange to meet a survivor who has already been in a group. You can talk together about what actually happens in the group, and the more experienced group member may be able to support you in getting to the first meeting.

In the Wakefield groups, there is no pressure to talk about what actually happened during the sexual abuse or who the abuser was. The initial emphasis is on how the abuse made the survivors feel about themselves and how it affects their lives now.

> We didn't give all the gory details of our abuse, we talked about the problems the abuse had left us with. I had forgotten so much about my own abuse but others in the group could remember and a lot of things they said prompted flashbacks and memories in me. **Jocelyn**

The group then moves on to understanding and expressing their feelings about the abuse and to working out ways of overcoming their current problems.

STICKING WITH IT

> In the first session, the therapists explained how we were likely to feel worse during the first few weeks as discussing the abuse made it more of a reality. It was only by revisiting the experiences that we could face up to our problems and overcome our bad feelings. This was very true. I soon began to feel the past feelings of shame and self-disgust and all the childhood experiences and emotions

came flooding back to me. Having been pre-warned about this was very helpful. **Eileen**

You may get to the first meeting but want to drop out after a few weeks. It's certainly not easy being in a survivors' group or in individual therapy. All the bad memories and unpleasant feelings that you have been trying to push to the back of your mind come to the surface. You need to face them again so you can accept them, share them, release the pain and power of the memories and start the healing process.

> During the group, you start thinking about your abuse all the time, when you're eating or cooking you're still thinking about it. You wake up in the night thinking about it again and you feel you should just hide it and try to forget about it again but you know you've got to get it out and deal with it, you can't hide it for ever.
>
> At first I thought, what have I done – I'm making things worse. I wished I'd never started. But now I realize I've got to get it out and face it and then maybe I can break free of it. I went through a phase of feeling really angry that I could have been so different if I hadn't been abused. It's been a horrible year. There was a lot to be uncovered and it wasn't nice. It's been very hard but I've got sorted out now. **Claire**

Here is what Pam's husband had to say.

> Eventually Pam got help at a survivors' group, but it didn't all end there. The more she went to the group for a while, the worse she became. For a few weeks there was no living with her. For two days after each group session, it was like living with a polecat with piles. I still cringe at the thought of those days.
>
> It was worth it though. Pam is certainly a different person now to the one who started going to the survivors' group. She still has some hang-ups but she is much more assertive and able in day-to-day life. **Brian**

There may be times when you want to give up and to blot it all out again. However, if you try to push your feelings down, they will surface again or come out in other ways such as anxiety, depression or eating problems. Talk about your feelings, and try to stick it out.

> It got a lot worse. It seems so long ago now since I've had a bad patch. But there were times when things were getting on top of me. It was triggering memories off that I brought home with me,

and were on my mind all the time. I was worse than before I went to the group. It seemed to last a long while but it was probably just three or four days solid. It was as if it was all fighting to come out and then it was all right. I rang my psychologist and said I didn't know if it was worth it but then I went back to the group and talked it through with them, that really helped. But I couldn't have stopped half-way through. I knew if I got there the first week that I would stick it out to the end. **Jocelyn**

HOW THE GROUP HELPED
In the rest of this section we look at what survivors found most helpful about being in a group.

Creating a safe environment

If I had to think of one thing that helped me in the group it would be honesty. I really believe throughout my life I haven't been honest with anybody and I felt in the group from the beginning that everyone wanted to be honest. We had all held a secret but it wasn't a secret in there. I could go in there and say anything, things I wouldn't have told anyone else, and I knew it was safe. **Jocelyn**

One of the most important things about a group is that it can create a safe environment where survivors can talk freely without putting on a brave face. They can talk honestly about their innermost fears and still feel respected and accepted by the other group members. This helps them to overcome the feelings of guilt and shame. They can also start to learn to trust others again.

When I was there in the group room I started to feel better but then I had to go home and cope with the outside world. Even though it was difficult, hard work and distressing, I felt secure there, even more so than in individual work with the therapist. **Colleen**

The group room was the first place that I know I could go to and be safe. The first time in my life I would feel that safety, that security, that peace, for which I had always been yearning and searching. I could go there to be among people I knew would accept me for *me*, not my act, not my front. I could relax with people for the very first time in my life. I felt comfortable and at home. The room was my place of security and it gave me the

courage to break free and be born again, totally free of guilt.
Clancy

Sharing feelings and being accepted

Before I joined the group, I tended not to think about things so
they wouldn't hurt as much. Getting things out in the open was
upsetting at the time but you need to do that to carry on and go
further. You think it's going to hurt too much to get things out
but it's worth it, even if it's difficult. I didn't realize how badly
it affected people; the women have done some awful things to
themselves and I think I've got away very mildly. But it's nice
to know the other people know what you're going through and
what you're thinking about. You feel you can trust them because
they've gone through it. **Claire**

In the group, survivors can share their feelings about themselves
and still feel accepted.

I always thought other people were judging me. In the group you
talk to other people who know exactly how you feel and accept
you. **Anita**

I found the group very helpful and I benefited enormously just
by being with other people who had had the same experiences as
me. I felt at ease with them. **Anthony**

I've only felt like me again since joining the group and getting
everything out and hearing others saying similar things. It's like
looking in a mirror. There's a feeling in the group that other people
are interested in what you've got to say. There wasn't an ulterior
motive to what people were saying or doing. A couple in my group
were very open and honest from the beginning, which made it
easier for me. We jelled quickly. I could never eat anything before
the group and after the group I could never go straight home.
      One day I went into the group and said it felt lighter in the
room and it was, as if everyone had suddenly unburdened themselves. We seemed to find each week, if you'd had a bad week
then the others had had similar experiences. We went through a
period where we all had a lot of nightmares or we were all angry
at our mothers. We could relate to each other so well. **Jocelyn**

The group helped because I knew I was not alone. I had time
to talk about myself. I felt respected even after I'd disclosed my
abuse and the group helped me realize it was not my fault. It also

helped to compare the way I'd coped with how the other men had coped. We acknowledged that each of us cope in different ways and we didn't judge each other negatively for turning to drink, drugs or self-harm. **Luke**

Talking to each other helps the survivors let go of some of their bad feelings.

I feel better when I come out of a group meeting. When I arrive I feel tense and a bit nervous but once I've left the group and I'm walking down the street I feel great. You have a chance to say what you feel. It's a way of releasing it. You may have been bottling it up all week but when you get to the group you can talk about it. **Mavis**

The survivors also learn to trust each other.

Most surprisingly the group became very close knit and extremely supportive to each other even during the first few weeks. There was a feeling of trust and a strong bond began to build up between us. This was extremely helpful as no one felt inhibited in discussing very deep and intimate problems. **Eileen**

They start to feel safe enough to allow their innermost feelings to surface and be expressed. Facing up to their feelings instead of blocking them off also helps them to feel less powerless and more in control.

As the group went on, I saw there was such a big change in me in the way I thought about myself. When things cropped up that I couldn't cope with, they supported and helped me. They didn't tell me what to do but they would give me ideas and we'd talk about it. I knew I'd got them supporting me and I wasn't alone, whereas before I'd always been alone. **Lucy**

Making the links

As long as I can remember I'd never liked myself, I was always moody, bad-tempered and angry. Since going to the group and letting my anger out I'm not like that any more. I realized I was angry for a reason. **Jocelyn**

Survivors grow up thinking of themselves as bad, mad or different from other people. As adults, they may still believe these things about themselves and so feel worthless and depressed. They often do not connect their present feelings and problems with their earlier abuse. In the group, they can see how the other group members have similar problems and begin to understand where their own problems come from.

> I didn't know my shaking had anything to do with my abuse.
> **Mavis**

> I kept telling myself I haven't been affected, I don't need to go to the group. But I'm glad I did, because as the group has gone on I've realized the abuse affected me more than I thought. At first I told myself I was just going along for Joan's sake (my sister), but I'm getting a lot out of it for myself. I can see how it's affected me now. I thought if you were sexually abused it only affected you in a relationship with another man, but it causes all sorts of problems. I'd never thought about that at all. **Claire**

> My abuse happened when I was about 7. I couldn't remember a lot. I thought it hadn't affected me because I couldn't remember what actually happened and it didn't go on for very long. But since being in the group I can see that I was riddled with guilt. You don't realize how much it has affected you until you get into a group and then you can see. It messed up 23 years of my life.
> **Jocelyn**

Making friends

> I couldn't wish for a better group. We're *friends* and see each other outside the group and ring each other up if we've got a problem or are worried about each other. **Lucy**

Sharing their feelings and being accepted by people who knew about their sexual abuse has helped survivors learn to trust each other and develop close friendships, often for the first time in their lives.

> I used to feel there wasn't any point in living at all. It's hard to feel that people like you if you don't really like yourself. I'm surprised how well we all got on in the group. It's been good to be able to get in touch with the group members between sessions, even though we didn't at the beginning. **Colleen**

> The girls in our group have become very close. When I come to the group, I look forward to seeing all the other girls and finding out how they've got on. The girls from another group came to

meet us. I noticed that they were very very close, like they'd known each other for years, like sisters. **Claire**

The relationship between survivors in a group is like that between men fighting a war in the trenches. They all have different personalities and different likes and dislikes. In the outside world they might never become friends, yet they have shared something that forms a bond. They have gone through hell together, fought side by side for every little victory one of them has achieved and picked each other up in their setbacks and defeats. The bond between men who have fought a war in the trenches will last long after peace has come for all of them. Similarly, the bond between survivors is still there, long after each one of us has built a new life and has found peace with herself at last. **Ingrid**

The survivors often stay friends after the group has ended.

I'm talking about not going to the self-help group any more but I do want to meet up and keep in touch with the other women because we have shared so much. **Jocelyn**

Helping others

Being in a group with other people who have had similar experiences not only helps survivors to understand their own problems, but also allows them to help other group members. Helping others, while respecting their own needs, can increase survivors' self-esteem and decrease their feelings of powerlessness.

It was definitely good to listen to other people and feel I could help. Giving support as well as receiving it gives you confidence, and helps you realize things about your own situation. **Colleen**

It also helped being able to help the others. You can understand how they feel, and talk about how you coped. Helping someone else made me feel better about myself. **Lucy**

Overcoming the problems

I've changed in so many ways I wouldn't have believed it. It would be nice if you could take a video at the beginning and end of the group to see the big difference in everybody because they've all changed so much. Other members of the group probably see you change a lot quicker than you do yourself. **Lucy**

How do people feel after they have been in individual therapy or in a survivors' group? How does it change them and their lives? Below we look at some of the changes in the Wakefield survivors.

Breaking free of the guilt and shame

> Sometimes I used to wonder if I would ever get over this feeling of guilt. Now I don't feel guilty about what happened – I can lay the blame at my stepfather's door. The group has been wonderful for me – I don't know what would have happened to me if I hadn't been referred to clinical psychology. **Jane**

> I used to cope by taking overdoses but since starting the group I no longer do that. I am not ashamed any more and I am no longer afraid of my abuser. I am now enjoying life to the full. **Anthony**

Understanding how an abuser plans and sets up the situation where he can abuse helps survivors put the responsibility for the abuse on to the abuser and in time break free from their own feelings of guilt.

> Meeting others who were also sexually abused as children took away the terrible isolation. For the first time, I talked to people who understood how I felt and why. When I listened to them I thought, 'They could not have stopped their abuser, why did I feel guilty all my life that I found no way to stop mine?' The shame and guilt began to go after our first group meeting. **Katarina**

Sharing their experiences with others and being accepted allow survivors to feel less ashamed and more able to talk without shame about their abuse to their friends and family.

> I was so frightened of anybody else finding out. Now I feel like I want to tell more people. **Claire**

> Sometime soon I'll tell my mum. Before I really worried about anyone knowing but now the world could know as long as it helped them and helped me. **Lucy**

Along with the decrease in the feelings of guilt and shame comes an increase in self-esteem: the survivors feel better about themselves as people and accept they have rights too.

> I feel better about saying what I think. It doesn't matter so much how people see me. I feel more confident that I am doing the

right thing. I hadn't realized how much time I spent trying to please people and ultimately not succeeding. I take more time now to stand back and assess situations rather than jumping in. **Jane**

Better relationships

I've got more confidence although I still have a way to go. I'm starting to get on with other people again. I'm going out a lot more. I never used to go out at all while my husband was working away. **Mavis**

I'm more open with people – I want to be friends now. **Jocelyn**

Therapy allows survivors to feel better about themselves and overcome their lack of trust. This enables them to begin forming relationships with other people. As we saw earlier, survivors who attended groups were also helped by forming close relationships within the group.

Before the group I was frightened of making relationships, and I thought that anyone who looked at me would know what had happened to me. I thought I was such a terrible person. I didn't want to go out before. It's nice now to go out socially. **Lucy**

Survivors learn to trust their therapist or each other first, and this gives them the courage to begin to develop other relationships. After working on their feelings towards their abusers, they can also improve their relationships with their sexual partners or begin to form new sexual relationships with people they can trust.

Lucy had been terrified of men, but after the group she became engaged and is now married and has a daughter.

Overcoming sexual problems

For years, I had sex promiscuously, fucking from the neck down, trading sex for a moment's attention, for a cuddle even. This was followed by several years of total dislike of sex after the birth of my first child. I gradually learned to share my feelings, fears and needs with my husband, and to help him share his with me. As we learned to communicate within other 'safe' areas of our relationship, to communicate with our hearts and minds, we were more able to communicate with our bodies. We learned to give each other privacy and to support one another. Gradually we were able to give one another the confidence we each needed to let ourselves be vulnerable. Sex can be about love and now for us it can be as free and liberated, as erotic or as close and comforting as we both want it to be. **Shirley**

Survivors often have sexual difficulties resulting from their earlier abuse. They can work on these problems with a therapist or in a group by learning to accept their bodies, to love and respect themselves and to trust and relate to other people. Survivors often do not know what is 'normal' sexually, and it can help to discuss this in a group and learn more about sex and sexuality.

Learning to enjoy sexual intimacy may not happen early in therapy because it is important to deal with issues relating to self-esteem, body image, trust in others and communication with your partner (if you have one) first. As Shirley's account shows, it *is* possible to overcome problems around sex and develop a close and loving sexual relationship.

Feeling powerful

Now I feel that I am in control. I know I still have weaknesses and I will continue to work on them. I am not a perfect person but I now acknowledge that I also have talents and a lot to offer. I am so thankful to Jehovah God that he has brought and directed me through the right channel so at last I can feel like me and know who I am. **Kate**

Having no control about what happens during sexual abuse often leaves survivors feeling powerless in their later lives and unsure who they are. During therapy, survivors learn to face up to their fears and overcome their feelings of powerlessness. Many return to work or start new jobs.

I packed my job in after I had a panic attack in the canteen. Before the group, I didn't think I would ever be able to get another job. I don't know when the change started, but near the end of the group I got a job working behind a bar. The first time I tensed up and began shaking, but the landlord said I did well. I enjoy it now, I feel better about myself since I started at the pub. **Mavis**

Releasing the tension that holds back the fears and becoming aware of their own worth and abilities often gives survivors renewed energy and a feeling that they can take control of their lives again. When you are worried and stressed, you have no energy.

Now I feel full of life and energy. I could conquer anything at the moment. I think much more of myself and have more confidence. I've got so many things I want to do now. I can't see I'll have time to fit everything in. I feel like making a fresh start. I want to go to the Technical College and do a course. **Claire**

Becoming aware of their own self-worth and learning to take control of their lives often helps survivors rid themselves of problems with drugs, alcohol or eating.

A lot of the problem was my weight and once I lost weight I felt a lot better about myself. But I could never have done it without the group. I began to feel I was worth something – that I had something to offer as a person. People were interested in me and I could have pride in myself. Before the group there didn't seem any point in losing weight and I was frightened of men so it worked in keeping them away. If I hadn't come to the group I would have lacked the confidence to say to myself: 'You're doing this for you because you want to lose weight and feel more confident.' **Colleen**

Assertion training or confidence-building helps survivors understand that they have rights and teaches how to express them. The feelings of powerlessness fade as survivors overcome their fears, understand why they felt so bad about themselves, and come to feel they can cope with their life and stand up for their rights.

Mainly I feel quite happy with myself and fairly confident. I'm trying to be assertive. Now I can give my opinion again. I feel as if I've got the vivacity that I had when I was 17. I feel like I can handle most situations. Obviously I have ups and downs, which is good – it's just like anybody else. **Colleen**

Finding yourself

I was so scared of the change, of letting go of my image, my 'front'. But I'm just me – released from the pain and guilt. It's so great just to feel comfortable with myself at last. **Clancy**

Talking about your sexual abuse, understanding and accepting what really happened and breaking free from your problems can release the person you are underneath. Instead of hiding behind the 'front' you present to the world, you can find your true self and live your life as you want to.

> Before I joined the survivors' group, I felt confused about who I was. Now through opening up, being honest, revealing the 'secret', I have found me, and I like what I am. I am not bad, inferior, a person of no importance, or worth. The anger and frustration and hate that I thought was me have been sorted out. It has been painful, it has been hard, but I was abused 23 years ago, and since then I have been living a lie. Now I feel free, free and lighter, I have been released. This 'secret' held me down and gradually over time it eventually dragged me down, but now it cannot hurt me any more. I have survived it. Now I can hold my head up, I don't have to pretend any more. I am not afraid, no one has a hold on me. The anger and frustration has gone; I feel happier, lighter, peaceful. It's the feelings inside me that have changed. I was always running away from *me* and I don't need to any more. I couldn't believe that just talking would help, it did, it does. I like myself, I did nothing wrong. **Jocelyn**

Suggestion

Your next step in overcoming problems resulting from sexual abuse may be to work through the exercises in the *Breaking Free Workbook*.

The progress of six of the survivors in this book is followed up, 7 years on, in Chapter 17, 'The journey continues'.

Reference

Pinnell, Sally (1989) 'An exploratory study of the process of change during group therapy for adult survivors of childhood sexual abuse', MSc dissertation in Clinical Psychology, Psychiatry and Behavioural Sciences, Leeds Institute of Health Sciences, Leeds.

16

Working towards prevention

In this chapter, we look at what you can do to help prevent the sexual abuse of children and young people. As we have seen, child sexual abuse is very common and is all around us; becoming aware of the widespread prevalence of sexual abuse can make you feel depressed and powerless. Taking action to help prevent further abuse can help you feel empowered again. It is possible for you to play an important part in the prevention of sexual abuse if you feel you want to.

Before you think about what you can do to help others, it is · important that you work through your feelings about your own abuse and overcome any problems the abuse has created in your life. You may want to put your energies into looking after and trying to protect other people, but *you* are important too. You deserve an opportunity to be yourself and be fulfilled in your own life. We recommend that you receive some help for yourself before you think about what you can do to help others. Some survivors move on to become counsellors and therapists and often do a great job helping clients who were sexually abused as children. It is especially important that survivors who work in the caring professions have resolved their own difficulties resulting from past abuse before they try to support others.

The spread of child sexual abuse

Child sexual abuse is a crime. Perpetrators abuse children and young people in secret and manipulate them into keeping quiet to enable their abuse to continue. This allows them to go on to abuse more and more children. Research and clinical work show that abusers can, and do, abuse many children and young people, sometimes over several decades.

Adults who were abused as children often end up feeling powerless. Some go on to form adult relationships with abusive people who physically, emotionally or sexually abuse them, and may also abuse their children. Survivors' own childhood experiences may leave them desperate to protect their own children but unable to *appropriately* protect them from abuse. A small number of sexually abused people do go on to abuse children themselves. Every abuser at loose in society can create a spreading wave of distress and further abuse.

How can we prevent sexual abuse?

To stop the spread of sexual abuse, we need to break the silence. For each child or adult survivor who can talk about his or her abuse, there is at least one abuser who can be prevented from harming other children. For each abuser who is prevented from having access to children, dozens of children could be protected from abuse and saved from years of suffering.

Children and young people who disclose and receive help need not go on to develop problems that last throughout their lives. Children who are believed and protected from further abuse need not carry forward the feelings of shame, self-blame, betrayal and powerlessness. Adults who disclose can receive help for themselves, overcome their feelings of powerlessness, and learn how to protect themselves and their own children from abuse.

We can all work towards the prevention of sexual abuse by: teaching children and young people how to protect themselves, looking out for signs of abuse and listening to children. It is possible to begin the process of prevention of sexual abuse at a grass-roots level by breaking the secret, talking about sexual abuse, encouraging people to listen to their children, learning ways to protect children and young people, and acting to prevent abusers from having access to children.

In this chapter, we suggest ways of responding to adults who choose to disclose their own experiences of childhood abuse to you. We describe how people can protect the children and young people in their care from sexual abuse, and how they should respond if they suspect abuse or if a child discloses to them. We also look at what you can do to prevent your own abuser, or any other abusers you are aware of, from having access to other children. The work Wakefield survivors have done towards prevention is described. The final section of the chapter looks at wider issues involved in the prevention of sexual abuse.

Listening to adults

After they have been through therapy, most of the Wakefield survivors begin to talk openly, and without any shame, about their own experiences of sexual abuse. Often the friends or other family members they have disclosed to tell them they have also been abused as children. In breaking your silence, you can help others to talk about their experiences, receive help and hopefully prevent further abuse. Listening to adult survivors who want to talk about their abuse is the first step in helping them break free from their pain and shame. It also means the survivors are more likely to learn how to appropriately protect their own children and save a new generation from experiencing abuse. The survivor may also act to prevent the perpetrator (or perpetrators) from harming other children and young people.

> I started talking among my friends and acquaintances about my own abuse and about the therapy I was receiving. More and more of them disclosed their own sexual abuse to me. Almost every one of my women friends has experienced some form of sexual abuse as a child. That was when I realized I could not remain silent. I remember too vividly my own despair when my need to be listened to and understood found nothing but deaf ears.
> **Ingrid**

What do you do if an adult discloses to you? The first thing to remember is that there is no need to panic and feel you have to do something straight away. A child who is being abused needs immediate protection, but with an adult survivor the abuse happened in the past. In some cases, the abuse may still be ongoing and the person will need support and acceptance until he or she is able to stop the abuse.

When people begin to talk about their own childhood abuse, all you need to do is listen, believe them and accept them. Let them tell you as much or as little as they want to. Make it clear you believe them. They may want to meet with you again to talk about it. Do not feel that you have to be responsible for the person, but do let them know they need to keep on talking about it, recommend they read this book or another book on recovering from the effects of sexual abuse and encourage them to get some professional help – see 'Sources of help' at the back of this book. **If the person(s) who has abused the adult has current access to children, protect the children by following the procedures below.**

Protecting children and young people

At least 10 per cent of children and young people are sexually abused. You can learn how to protect children around you from abuse and how to support children and young people who have already been abused. Each child that you help in this way can be saved from a lifetime of problems. If it leads to the identification of another abuser, it can also be a step towards the prevention of the abuse of other children. A few abused children and young people will begin to act out the abuse with other children and may eventually become perpetrators themselves; receiving help straight away for the effects of the abuse they have themselves experienced can stop the cycle of abuse from repeating itself.

The only certain way to prevent children from being abused is to ensure they are not available to an abuser. Children and young people are sexually abused because an abuser has access to them, not because of anything that the child does. Children should never be left alone, even briefly, with anyone who is known, or suspected, to be an abuser.

In this section, we will look at how you can watch for signs of abuse in children and young people, how you can encourage a child to disclose abuse to you, what to do if a child does disclose to you and how you can teach children to protect themselves.

SIGNS OF ABUSE/'SILENT WAYS OF TELLING'
Children and young people often show they are in distress by changes in their behaviour. Finding out why they are behaving 'badly', or differently from usual, may uncover sexual abuse or other difficulties they are struggling with. You can encourage children and young people to talk about how they are feeling and what is disturbing them, and give them an opportunity to disclose any abuse.

Many children who are being sexually abused do not tell anyone what is happening to them, but they may show that they are in distress, or give signs that they are being abused. They may start bedwetting, have nightmares, become withdrawn, have stomach aches or become clingy or aggressive. Some of these signs are described in Box 4 in Chapter 5. It is important to know that children who show these signs are not necessarily being sexually abused. The behaviour changes could be caused by some other disturbance in their lives, such as a divorce or death in the family, bullying at school or physical or emotional abuse.

Sexual abuse may be suspected if a child has more sexual knowledge than you would expect for his or her age, or is acting in a sexually inappropriate way. The concerned adult needs to find out where and how the child accessed the sexual information. It may have been through sexual abuse, but it may have been from exposure to sexual activity on the television, or from accessing sexual material or pornography on the internet.

Disturbed behaviour indicates that something is wrong, and the child or teenager needs a trusted adult to try to find out what is happening to him or her. A child or teenager having money or gifts that they cannot account for could also be a sign that they are being groomed for abuse or are receiving rewards for being involved in sexual activity from a perpetrator or group of perpetrators. If you are concerned about a child, ask for advice from the NSPCC or other helpline and encourage the young person to talk to you. You could also provide the young person with websites or phone numbers for helplines that he or she could contact directly.

LISTENING TO CHILDREN AND YOUNG PEOPLE

To encourage your children to talk to you, show them you have time for them and want to listen to them. Make sure they know you will protect them, and not punish them, if they tell you about any inappropriate sexual behaviour they have experienced or heard about. Children may not talk about the abuse directly. They may say, 'I don't like Mr Brown' or 'I don't want to stay at Grandad's any more.' Try not to dismiss what they say. Find out more: ask them why they don't like that person, or why they don't want to stay somewhere or go out with someone. If a child feels uncomfortable with someone, respect their feelings. If you are receptive, your child will be more likely to talk.

This is Kate's advice on how to protect your children.

Talk to and listen to your children. Their feelings count. If they don't like someone's company ask yourself 'Why?' Don't force them to go with people they don't like, dismissing it by saying they're awkward or playing up. Don't put children down by calling them a baby if they are afraid of something or someone. If boys or girls are afraid there's a reason – find it out. Believe your children. Don't dismiss their worries or fears or dislikes. **Kate**

What do you do if your child (or another child or young person) tells you he or she has been sexually abused?

- Don't panic. Try not to show how upset or angry you are.
- Listen to him or her.
- Believe the child, and let the child know you believe him or her.
- Tell the child that he or she is right to tell you, and don't blame the child in any way (for example, by saying 'Why didn't you tell me before?')
- Tell him or her you will not let it happen again. Make sure the child is not left alone with the abuser however briefly.
- Tell the child you may need to tell someone else to get help to protect him or her. Explain to the child what you are going to do and why, and try not to let the child feel they have no control over what is going to happen next. Inform the local authority child protection team (see below).
- Do not threaten to kill or harm the abuser. This may make the child feel guilty or frightened. Let the child know it doesn't matter what the child did, or any rewards he or she might have accepted, the abuser is always responsible for the abuse.
- Make sure the child gets some help to work through his or her confused feelings about the abuse. Ask your GP to refer the child to an appropriate agency, such as clinical psychology or the Child and Adolescent Mental Health Service (CAMHS) or contact social services or the NSPCC.

If a child does disclose to you, you will probably feel upset, angry or shocked. Try to get some support for yourself. Remember that with appropriate help now, the child will not necessarily develop immediate or long-term problems.

When I began to talk freely about sexual abuse, my daughter had the confidence to tell me that it had happened to her three years previously when she was five years old. Because she could tell me so early in life, and because I know what help she needs to overcome her shame and guilt, I know that she will grow up without the mental scars that a continued silence would have produced. **Ingrid**

TEACHING CHILDREN AND YOUNG PEOPLE HOW TO PROTECT THEMSELVES

It is very difficult to identify an abuser unless you know they have abused a child. They don't look any different from anyone else and outwardly may appear to be very nice, respectable members of the community. You cannot be with your children 24 hours a day for the rest of their lives, so it is important to teach children and young people how to recognize situations that are dangerous or simply difficult or uncomfortable.

I don't want to frighten my child

Many people are worried that, by teaching children and young people about the dangers of sexual abuse, they will make them frightened and mistrustful of all adults. This is an understandable worry, but if the subject is approached in the right way it does not need to be a problem. We do not need to teach children to fear and distrust people; we can teach them positive skills to help them feel safe. We can teach them that their bodies belong to themselves and they don't have to let anyone touch their body in a way they don't like.

We teach children how to cross the road and protect themselves from the dangers of traffic without making them terrified of cars or too fearful to ever step off the pavement. We can also teach children how to protect themselves from sexual abuse without making them fearful of every adult.

What to teach your children

You need to teach your children that they have the right to feel safe and that they can talk to you openly, whatever happens to them. Tell them you will believe them and not be angry with them if they tell you about being touched or feeling uncomfortable with someone. Encourage them to trust their own instincts and listen to their own bodies if they feel uncomfortable with anyone. Teach them that their bodies belong to them and they have the right to say 'No'. Show them you mean this, by giving them choice about physical contact. Ask them if they want to give you or anyone else a kiss or cuddle but do not insist. It may be embarrassing if your children refuse to kiss someone, but support them if they do this. Explain to your friends and relatives that your children have the right to choose who they kiss and cuddle.

Teach children the difference between surprises, like birthday presents and parties, and secrets. Tell them they should not keep secrets, even if they are told to, and that they can talk to you or another trusted adult if anyone asks them to keep a secret. Make it clear to children that the rules apply to everyone, including family members.

You can also teach them general safety rules about not talking to strangers and not going into other people's homes without permission, for example. It will be easier for them to talk about sexual abuse if they know the words for body parts and sexual acts. Teach them some basic sex education. Make clear the difference between sexual assault and consensual sex, so they do not grow up afraid of appropriate sexual activity.

Remember that young children take what you say literally. Be as clear as you can and check that the child has understood you correctly.

> When I was very small my mum told me not to take sweets from strangers. I thought this was because they might be poisoned. When an old lady on a bus offered us some sweets and my mum said it was all right to have one, I was really impressed that my mum could tell who had poisoned sweets and who hadn't.
> **Shirley**

You can start to teach very young children about protecting themselves at a level they can understand. Show them they have rights by giving them choices about physical contact, and in other ways like allowing them to choose which book to read at bedtime or which clothes to wear. Play 'What if . . .' games, with questions such as 'What would you do if the babysitter asks you to keep a secret?' Keep talking to your children about protecting themselves – don't just do it once. There are many good books available on how to protect children.

Protecting young people – the internet and social media

As soon as children are old enough to have their own smartphones or have unsupervised access to the internet via computers or other devices, they need to be informed about the increasing range of dangers associated with the internet and social media platforms. It is the parents' responsibility to restrict the child's access to sexually explicit online material that is not appropriate for the age of the child, as well as warning them of the harm that viewing pornography can do to them.

Seeing any form of pornography invites a young person to compare their own bodies, genitals and possibly sexual performance in a negative way with the actors or victims involved in the videos or photographs. Viewing extreme pornography can traumatize a young person as well as possibly being harmful to the 'actors' involved and could be illegal; this is especially true of child pornography, which is illegal and is definitely harmful to the child victims depicted.

Sexting (texting explicit sexual material) and sending photographs of themselves naked or in sexual poses are common among young people. The young people may believe they can trust the boyfriend or girlfriend they send the messages to, but afterwards the text, photos or videos are sometimes shared on social media ('revenge porn'), causing shame and distress to the victim. Children and young people can be groomed via social media, chat rooms or other digital platforms by an older person who pretends to be another young person (posing as a friend, or a boyfriend or girlfriend). They may be persuaded to send naked or sexual 'selfies' that can then be used to blackmail the young person into meeting up with the potential abuser, or into sexual activities they do not consent to.

Tens of thousands of people in this country download indecent images of children every year. Unfortunately, a fifth of the indecent images of children uploaded to the internet are taken by the children themselves. It is important for parents, and others who are responsible for children, to educate them about the consequences of sending any explicit material to others, however much the young people feel they trust them at the time, and to make sure that the young people know that they will lose all control of how widely that information can be disseminated.

Young people should also be aware that any material (including photos, videos and text) that is uploaded to the internet in any form (for example, via social media platforms, chat forums, photo apps and so on) will be digitally stored for ever and can still be available for viewing in the future. This applies even after you have deleted information from view and also applies when you use apps where the information is only displayed for a short time before disappearing – it is still stored and accessible.

Some of the Wakefield survivors drew up a list of things you can teach your children and young people to keep them safe from abuse. This is shown in Box 10.

Stopping the abusers

Now I'm questioning myself as to whether or not I should do something about the abuser, to put a stop to it all, to protect my own daughter and other children in the family. If he died I wouldn't have all these decisions to make. I ought to do something about it, but can I? Am I letting my own daughter down if I don't? What would it achieve anyway? One year in prison, then out. Could I be the one to put him in prison? Perhaps he would die in prison. He would certainly suffer, but I don't want him to suffer even though it would be his fault because he's an abuser. I would still feel responsible. But then I would feel responsible if he abuses anyone else. It could be partly my fault if he abuses any more children because I didn't do anything. But how could I hurt my mum? **Kate**

Deciding to take action about your abuser can be a very difficult decision to make. Kate was racked with indecision. Her father had abused her and her nine brothers and sisters, his grandchildren, nieces and many others. She didn't want to hurt her father or her mother by exposing his activities, but she couldn't sit back and let him abuse even more children. (Kate and her sister did confront their father to prevent him abusing even more family members – see Chapter 14 for more of their story.)

Abusers may abuse dozens of children throughout their lifetime and often continue abusing into their old age. After group therapy, survivors begin to talk about their abuse to their friends and family and often find some of them have been abused by the same abuser.

Box 10 Teaching your children to feel safe

Teach them (choose the items that are appropriate to the age of the child):

- that they have the right to feel safe and they should tell someone if anyone makes them feel afraid or uncomfortable;
- that if a person touches them in a way they don't like or if they feel uncomfortable or uneasy about anything, they should tell an adult they trust and if that person doesn't believe them or help them, they should tell someone else and keep telling until someone does help;
- that the rules apply to everyone, including family members, teachers, babysitters, religious leaders and so on;
- that they should think of five people they can trust (family members, teacher and so on) who they could approach if they have any concerns;
- that you will believe them and not be angry if they tell you of an incident when they have been touched or felt uncomfortable or if they have broken any of the rules about keeping safe;
- not to keep secrets (but not telling about surprises, such as presents and parties, is OK);
- that they are allowed to disobey an adult if they are in danger or to protect themselves – it's OK not to be polite in order to protect themselves;
- how to say 'NO', shout 'STOP' and run away;
- the difference between good touch and bad touch – bad touch is anything that makes them feel uncomfortable, confused or uneasy;
- what their private parts are (their private parts are covered by a swimsuit, so their breasts, buttocks, genitals) and no one should touch their private parts, unless the person is a doctor or a nurse and their mother or father is with them (it's OK for them to touch themselves);
- they should not touch the private parts of another child or an adult;
- that they have the right to say 'NO' if anyone touches them in a way they don't like or makes them feel uncomfortable – they don't have to kiss or cuddle anyone, young or old, if they don't want to and they have a right to say who touches them and how – and they can say, 'It's my body – I decide';
- about the dangers of interacting with people they don't know online or on any social media platform – they should never arrange to meet anyone they have met online and should tell

---

you or a trusted adult if they have any concerns about any online interactions;

- that they should not be persuaded to post any photos of themselves naked or in sexual postures – these photos can be widely shared and will always exist online;
- not to talk to strangers who approach them or go anywhere with strangers;
- to tell an adult, even a stranger, if they think they are being followed or believe they are in danger;
- to be wary of special favours and bribes and blackmail;
- that it's OK to ask about other people's puzzling or confusing behaviour, such as, 'Why does Uncle George want to play the funny game?';
- how to use the telephone and memorize their own telephone number and that of a trusted person;
- rules about being invited into another person's home when playing out;
- a password that can be used if an unfamiliar person has to collect them from school;
- about the dangers of sexual exploitation, such as being manipulated into sexual relationships and rewarded with gifts, affection, praise and so on, and that an older person may deceive the young person by pretending to be a boyfriend/girlfriend in order to involve the young person in a sexual relationship with him or her and possibly, later on, with a gang of other abusers;
- warnings about how drugs and alcohol can be used to manipulate them into sexual relationships;
- about sex education and the difference between consensual sex and sexual assault;
- that young people should put the registration number of any taxi they use into their phones – they can then send you a text message if they have any concerns about the taxi driver;
- that young people should send a text message or phone if they are concerned about anything that is happening to them or their friends when out at night – this could be a prearranged code.

Forty per cent of the Wakefield survivors know of at least one other child who was abused by the same abuser as themselves. Abusers keep on scheming, planning and creating opportunities to abuse more children and young people.

WHAT CAN YOU DO ABOUT IT?

Child sexual abuse is happening all around us. To protect the next generation, we must act every time we have any suspicions. What can you do to prevent your abuser from abusing other children? The most important thing is to ensure that abusers do not have access to any children and young people. If you have children, talking about your awareness of sexual abuse to your circle of friends and acquaintances may warn off any potential abusers.

Children at risk

You will rarely be certain that your abuser is still abusing. If your abuser (or another abuser you know of) has children of his or her own, or has access to children, these children are at risk and you should inform the local authority child protection team, whether or not you know for certain that he or she is abusing them. Child welfare is the responsibility of the local authorities, and they have a duty to investigate if there is reason to suspect a child is suffering, or likely to suffer, significant harm. The local authority will then investigate the situation and check all records (including those of the GP, health visitor or school) on any children involved. They will inform the police if they think any criminal activity is occurring. The priority, for all agencies involved, will be the welfare of the child.

Reporting suspected sexual abuse

If you know, or have strong suspicions, that a child is currently being abused, inform the local authority child protection team, the police (ask for the child abuse investigation unit) or the NSPCC immediately. If you can, provide them with the names and dates of birth of both the child and the abuser, and as much other information as you can. Give your own name if you can. This will be kept confidential and not given to the abuser or his or her family. You can make a report anonymously by telephone or letter, but then you will not be able to provide any further information that might be needed. If you work for an organization, make sure you are aware of, and follow, their child protection policy.

The child protection and criminal investigations will usually happen at the same time. Social services, health authorities, voluntary groups and the police now work together in the best interests of children, and their priority is to protect children from any form of abuse. At the very least, telephone one of the helplines given in the 'Sources of help' section at the back of this book and discuss the problem with them (the NSPCC is recommended).

If the child is in any immediate danger, phone the police (on 999) straight away.

Confronting abusers

In some cases, the abuser is still around but there are no children and young people in his or her immediate circle. In this circumstance, some of the Wakefield survivors decided to confront their abusers to let them know they were being watched; and to tell them they were warning people with children by informing them of the abusers' past sexual offences. *DO NOT* confront your abuser in person without fully preparing yourself as described in Chapter 14, 'Abusers'.

Prosecuting your abuser(s), and historical sex offences

Some adult survivors, like Joanne in Chapter 14, give statements to the police and attempt to prosecute their abusers to prevent them from abusing other children. In criminal law, it is the police and the courts who prosecute offenders (including those who sexually abuse children) to protect the public.

In England, Wales and Northern Ireland, there is no time limit on when you can prosecute for a major crime such as sexual assault of a child. Nowadays, anyone reporting historic sexual abuse to the police will be treated seriously and the case properly investigated. Because of the passage of time, there are likely to be difficulties in finding enough supporting evidence for the case to go to court. If the police find enough corroborating evidence, they will pass the file to the Crown Prosecution Service, which will decide whether or not to prosecute. This will depend on whether it is considered to be in the public interest and whether there is enough evidence for a reasonable chance of a conviction. The legal process can take a very long time (sometimes years) and have an uncertain outcome. Attending court can itself be very stressful.

If you want to consider prosecuting your abuser, please talk to a

professional (for example, Victim Support on 0808 168 9111 or visit
<www.victimsupport.org.uk>) about it first or phone the police and
discuss it with someone from the police child protection investigation unit. You can ask to speak to a policewoman, if this is what you
would prefer. They will explain the whole process to you, and you
can then decide if you want to go ahead.

From Report to Court is a very useful handbook that takes you
through all the steps from reporting abuse to going through the
court system (available online, see the 'Sources of help' section at
the back of the book for details).

Look in the 'Sources of help' section at the back of the book for
contact details and websites where you can find information about
the legal process.

ACT (ABUSE – COUNSELLING AND TRAINING)

Wakefield survivors have helped in the prevention of further
sexual abuse by breaking the secrecy around their own abuse, by
protecting any children and young people around them and by
ensuring the abusers do not harm any more children. Some of the
Wakefield survivors wanted to do more than this and formed an
action group called ACT, which aimed to help other people who
have been abused and to do further work towards the prevention
of abuse. The ACT members attended counselling courses themselves, counselled other survivors and worked towards increasing
public awareness of child sexual abuse. Being sexually abused can
make you feel helpless and out of control; ACT members found that
working towards the prevention of further abuse helped them feel
more powerful.

Working with survivors

> There are so many women who need help, too many women still
> in isolation, feeling they are the only ones. I gladly picked up the
> suggestion by the psychologists to meet some of the women who
> were on their waiting lists. Before therapy starts many survivors
> feel the stigma of shame and guilt very strongly and it helps
> them to meet another survivor who has been through therapy
> and will not only understand them but also reassure them that
> life will be so much better after receiving the help they so des-
> perately seek.

Many survivors hate themselves before they receive therapy. Meeting someone and liking someone who had the same experience of being abused makes it easier for them to begin to like themselves. **Katarina**

ACT members met with survivors who had been referred to Wakefield Clinical Psychology Service to talk to them about their own experiences and how it is possible to overcome the problems created by childhood abuse. The first groups were for female survivors, but these were quickly followed by groups for men and then mixed groups for male and female survivors. Some ACT members ran self-help groups for survivors.

We set up a survivors' Support Group. Initially this was an idea Lucy and I had, to help one survivor overcome her fear of groups. We started with just two survivors and every week added one more of the new survivors who were waiting for the next therapy group. Slowly they got used to each other, slowly they lost the fear of a group, although at times it still came back. They now talk openly about the effects of the abuse and are able to encourage the new survivors who still have to overcome their insecurities about being in a group. **Katarina**

ACT members attended some of the survivors' group sessions run by the psychologists. They encouraged group members to continue when they became distressed because they were facing up to their memories and feelings. ACT members gave the group members hope that recovery was possible, and they also attended sessions on specific topics to contribute their experiences and talk about how they had learnt to cope with the problems.

ACT members were also brave enough to get involved in several therapy groups for perpetrators – providing the abusers with a victim's perspective on abuse and strongly challenging the abusers' beliefs and excuses. They also ran crèches for the children of other survivors so they could attend a therapy group, worked as volunteers at a local domestic violence resource and drop-in centre, and met with and advised other groups of survivors from around the country. In addition, they were involved in campaigning for greater awareness and the prevention of sexual abuse by giving newspaper, radio and television interviews and by contributing to this book. ACT had an important role to play in helping many survivors in the local community who had just come forward for help or who were thinking about coming forward for help, and in reducing the amount of suffering that abuse causes.

You may want to join or set up a group to work towards prevention but do not feel you have to do this. Some survivors benefit from the therapy groups and afterwards just want to get on with their lives. They deserve to be able to put their past behind them at last and to fulfil their lives in whichever way they choose.

Recovered memories and 'false memory syndrome'

In the 1990s, there was much inaccurate and misleading information in the media about 'false memory syndrome'. Some survivors were told that they had not actually been sexually abused, but were suffering from 'false memory syndrome'; this increased the fears of other survivors that they would not be believed if they disclosed their own childhood abuse.

'False memory syndrome' is not actually a syndrome or a medical diagnosis. It is a term that was first used by the False Memory Syndrome Foundation in America in 1991. They used the term to describe people who had *not* been sexually abused somehow coming to believe that they had been abused, and creating memories of events in their childhood that had not occurred. Therapists were accused of inducing these 'false memories' in clients who came into therapy with no memories of childhood sexual abuse.

The term 'false memory syndrome' should *not* be applied to people who have actually been abused, and it does not apply to people who have always had some memories of their abuse. 'False memory syndrome' also does not describe people who knowingly make false accusations of abuse. False allegations of abuse can be made, but they are only a very small percentage of the allegations made, and false allegations do not occur any more often with child sexual abuse than with other crimes.

Some people take the view that it is not possible to forget about childhood abuse and therefore believe that anyone who recovers memories of abuse must have 'false memories'. There is a great deal of clinical evidence to support the fact that people can dissociate from traumas, including childhood sexual abuse, and have the memories re-surface later on in life. As we have previously discussed, memories of childhood sexual abuse can be triggered by events such as the birth of a child or the death of an abuser.

Survivors sometimes do recover memories of abuse while in therapy, perhaps because their memories have been triggered by talking about their childhoods, or because they feel safe enough with their therapist to allow the memories back into awareness. Recovering memories of abuse does not mean the memories are false. However, therapists cannot say how accurate these memories are, and they cannot diagnose sexual abuse from a person's symptoms. All memories can be distorted, so recovered memories, nightmares and flashbacks are not necessarily accurate recollections of the past.

There may be other information (for example, siblings may have witnessed the abuse or been abused by the same person) that can be used to corroborate the accuracy of memories, but some people with recovered memories may never know for sure what has happened to them.

To be falsely accused of abusing a child must be terrible; we need to be aware that this does *occasionally* happen, and we must do our best to prevent it. However, accusing their victims of having 'false memory syndrome' can also be an ideal defence for people who *have* sexually abused children. We hope this information will increase understanding and thereby encourage survivors to continue to speak out.

Wider issues in prevention

This chapter has looked at some of the ways you can work towards the prevention of sexual abuse. Why is the sexual abuse of children and young people so widespread? Why is it mostly men who abuse? These are questions that need to be addressed if we are to create a society that is safe for children. We can begin to try to answer these questions by looking at wider issues such as the general treatment of children and women in our society, the different expectations for males and females, and the effects of pornography.

In our society, children are devalued. Emotional, verbal, physical and sexual abuse of children is a daily occurrence. Children are powerless, and some adults feel it is acceptable to exert their power and control over children and young people in whatever way they want to.

There are many differences in the ways that boys and girls are brought up. Girls learn that, to be valued, they must be nurturing to others and not express anger. Girls and women who are victimized therefore usually turn their anger and distress in on themselves and become depressed, self-destructive and vulnerable to further abuse. Boys learn that, to be valued, they must appear to be powerful and not show any weakness. Boys and men who are victimized are more likely to turn their anger and distress outwards and try to regain their power by victimizing others, particularly those they see as less powerful than themselves. This means that men are more likely than women to become abusers.

Women have less access than men to money, jobs and influence. However, women are the ones who usually shoulder the emotional, practical and financial burden of childcare. The lack of legal protection afforded to women and children, and the lack of access to money, housing, childcare facilities and so on, put some women in a position where they may be powerless and vulnerable. This makes it difficult for these women to leave men who are violent or sexually abusive to themselves or their children.

Pornography, 'page three girls', 'trolling' women who speak out on social media and the use of women's bodies in advertising contribute to a climate in which women are not respected and are seen as sex objects. Child pornography (which is illegal) encourages abusers to believe it is normal and acceptable to have sex with children and young people. Pornography, especially child pornography, is used by abusers to fantasize about abuse, and this helps them to rationalize their abuse and believe they are doing no wrong. All kinds of pornography are easily accessible via the internet, and there need to be strong appropriate restrictions on the sites involved. It is also the case that people involved in uploading, maintaining or accessing sites where illegal material is available should be prosecuted.

Having sex with children and young people in other countries on sex tourism trips also encourages the belief that the sexual abuse of children is acceptable; people who engage in this activity should be also prosecuted.

We can begin to address these issues by making changes at an individual level in terms of how we relate to others and how we bring up children.

We can all play a small part in reshaping a society in which it is possible for children to be abused and for women to be regarded as of less importance than men. Each individual, whether she has been a victim of abuse or not, can try to influence those people close to her. It is not just the work of feminist movements or psychologists writing books and giving lectures. Parents can teach their sons to respect girls as equals and that it is not unmanly to show care, concern, sensitivity and understanding towards others, male and female alike. They can teach their sons and daughters to value their own rights and the rights of others. Women in the workplace can begin to put a stop to being treated as nothing more than ornaments who are not to be taken seriously. Wives can insist on being treated as having equal rights. Daughters can insist on being listened to in their wishes and plans for their own future. **Ingrid**

There is also a need for change in government policies and provision of resources. The impact of sexual abuse costs the UK billions of pounds in medical, mental health and social care every year, money that would be far better spent on the prevention of sexual abuse.

All abused children and adults need immediate help to overcome problems arising from sexual abuse. All professionals who work with children and young people should be trained to recognize the signs of abuse and how to deal with disclosures. Schools should teach children assertion skills and how to protect themselves from abuse. All abusers need treatment to confront them with the damage they are inflicting on others, to help them to overcome their motivation to abuse children and to stop them continuing to abuse children. It is particularly important for children who are victimizing other children to receive immediate therapy and understanding, to prevent them embarking on a lifetime of abusing others.

Summary

We can all play an important part in the struggle towards the prevention of sexual abuse. Just as individual abusers can set off a spreading wave of sexual abuse and distress, the fight against sexual abuse can spread out from individuals who are aware and want to keep children and young people safe. You can empower yourself, and help in the prevention of sexual abuse, by listening to and helping children and adults who have been abused, by learning how to help children remain safe and by ensuring your own abuser does not harm any other children and young people. You can make changes in your own life in the way you treat children and allow yourself to be treated. On a wider scale, people can organize to campaign for more resources for the treatment of victims and abusers, and to control pornography and material that degrades women and children.

The UK has been shocked by recent revelations of the widespread sexual abuse of children and other vulnerable people, over several decades, by celebrities, politicians and figures in positions of power. Many people who worked alongside these abusers, or suspected the abuse was happening, turned a blind eye. These scandals have massively increased the awareness of the general public and the authorities to the disturbing extent of child sexual abuse, how it can occur in plain sight and the lasting harm caused to the survivors.

The uncovering of these notorious crimes resulted in a major shake-up in the police service and in other authorities involved in child protection. Police officers are now trained in awareness of child sexual abuse, how to respond to victims coming forward and the importance of a thorough investigation. Police forces are coordinated at a national level to investigate non-recent child sexual abuse by prominent figures involving thousands of survivors.

The lesson we hope the general public and the authorities have learnt from the uncovering of these scandals is that we *all* need to act, *every* time we have any suspicions of child abuse. Survivors have suffered in silence for too long. Now it is time to speak out and protect the next generation of children. Breaking the silence helps you break free from the influence of your past abuse, takes power away from the abuser and can also help reshape a society where children are respected and sexual abuse is no longer common.

Suggestions

- It is important that you address your own emotions and difficulties before you try to help others, so do go for help if you haven't already done so. If you feel you want to work towards the prevention of further sexual abuse, follow the suggestions in the chapter.

- If you know or suspect that a child or young person is currently being abused, act immediately by following the instructions given in this chapter on how to protect them. Look for signs of abuse in children, and listen to children and young people who try to talk about their abuse. Teach your children how to protect themselves from abuse.
- Follow the suggestions given in the chapter to ensure your abuser, and any other abusers you become aware of, are not able to harm other children and young people.
- The 'Sources of help' section at the back of the book has information about who to contact if you have any worries about child protection. You will also find details of the website for Child Exploitation and Online Protection (CEOP), which you can contact if you have any concerns about online activity or child sexual exploitation.

Breaking Free in the NHS

The project described below is a step forward in helping survivors who have entered the mental health services to disclose any childhood sexual abuse that may be contributing to their current symptoms and mental health problems. The mental health service staff are trained to give every person being assessed an opportunity to talk about any childhood sexual abuse.

The Department of Health and National Institute of Mental Health in England (NIMHE) led an implementation process, involving all NHS mental health provider trusts, to establish the routine enquiry of abuse in mental health assessments and to ensure that survivors/victims receive the care and support they need following disclosures, through care-planning processes.

To equip staff to undertake routine enquiry and better meet the needs of the victims/survivors in their care – particularly those who have endured child sexual abuse – they received a 1-day sexual abuse training course. Integral parts of this training are the *Breaking Free* and *Breaking Free Workbook* publications. Each trust, as part of the project, is given one copy of each publication with a recommendation that trusts purchase these publications for every inpatient unit and community-based mental health team within their remit.

17

The journey continues

How we are now

Many survivors wonder whether they will ever overcome the impact of the sexual abuse on their lives or if they will always have problems and be haunted by their past. Others wonder if the progress they have already made will continue or if they will slip back to where they were. We have already seen how the survivors in this book began their journey to healing. Six survivors who contributed to the first edition of this book tell us about their current lives and the changes they have made. All six survivors were in group therapy. Ingrid, Kate, Fiona, Jane, Eileen and Pam tell us what they have been doing since therapy and how they are now.

Ingrid

Ingrid was sexually abused by her brother. She has now put the past behind her and has completely changed her life.

It is now more than a decade since I had therapy and my life could not be more different from before I joined the survivors' group. My confidence has improved greatly as has my ability to think positively. I no longer expect bad things to happen to me and no longer think that anything negative that happens to others is my fault.

I found the strength to divorce my husband after 14 years and leave a loveless and empty marriage. Finally free from restrictions I took a degree course with the Open University and studied psychology for 6 years. After receiving my degree I started a further degree course in philosophy and am now in my third year. After 14 years with my ex-husband as a housewife with small part-time jobs, I returned to the work force, working first as a secretary and later as office manager. I bought an old house and started to rebuild my life completely.

My life is very happy and fulfilled now. I will get married in 3 weeks and know this time the marriage will last. We have a partnership of equals in which not only love, but also respect, friendship and mutual consideration for each other's needs are important. Before therapy I would not have been able to have a relationship like this, as I did not feel equal to anybody.

I no longer have sexual problems but thoroughly enjoy the physical side of my relationship. Being touched and touching my partner does not bring on memories of abuse any more. I feel a freedom within me to do what I want and to be anything I want to be. I have learnt to love my body and myself and am happy to be me. **Ingrid**

Kate

Kate was sexually abused by her father (who sexually abused dozens of other family members) and other relatives. She has overcome the effects of the abuse and done everything she can to prevent further abuse within her own extended family and elsewhere.

I have worked in residential care and on projects. I have done my RSA in counselling skills. I have told my mother about the abuse and so no longer need to protect her. I have also confronted a paedophile who married into the family. I am no longer a Jehovah's Witness and actually view the six years that I was as quite an unhappy time of my life. When I reflect back, I realize that I was treated kindly by a few but unkindly by others. I strongly feel that I was robbed of my feelings and made to feel unworthy by some of them, and I was not taken note of when child protection issues arose. I now feel healed, loved, worthy and myself. **Kate**

Fiona

Fiona experienced a childhood of neglect and emotional, physical and sexual abuse within the family, and was sexually abused by many other perpetrators from outside the family. She had no opportunities as a child and had had little education. Fiona was barely literate when she came into therapy, but she worked hard to overcome the effects of the deprivation and abuse she had suffered and has now managed to create the life she wanted for herself.

I am a qualified trainer and I have gained my postgraduate diploma in counselling. I have continued to help other survivors by facilitating a support group. I have learnt to drive, which for me was a great achievement due to my earlier phobia. I also practise karate and have reached my brown belt (3rd Kyu). My relationship with my daughter is good. I do not overprotect her and she has appropriate freedom in terms of relationships (boyfriends). Relationships are better. I no longer use sex as a coping strategy. I am more assertive, I manage my anger well and I am a calmer person. I no longer have any obsessional behaviours or anxieties. I feel strong and can face anything. **Fiona**

Jane

Jane was sexually abused for 10 years by her stepfather. She has turned her life around, and now approaches her life from a position of strength, while accepting there will always be challenges to face.

Professionally I have taken on projects that I am interested in and that are fulfilling. I have been able to say what I am unable to take on and ask for support when I feel I need it. I am in a successful relationship with a man who says he enjoys being with an assertive woman and I believe him. We are happy in a relationship which is sharing, caring and supportive. We don't live together, choosing to respect each other's space and acknowledge our respective children's needs. I am surviving being a parent although I find my role as a parent most challenging. It is difficult to maintain secure boundaries and confidence when dealing with a teenage daughter who struggles with being assertive.

I am much more self-aware and can cope with experiences, feelings and situations much better. I know what will help me cope if I feel I need assistance. I feel confident and assertive. I am comfortable with myself and can give myself permission to make mistakes. Without the healing, I wouldn't have achieved any of this. **Jane**

Eileen

Eileen was sexually abused for much of her childhood by her uncle. She pursued a successful professional career for many years and is now able to use her retirement to further her skills and self-development. When we first met her, Eileen said she hoped that one day she would find 'the real me'.

> I am more positive about what I want in life, and no longer live in a soap opera where I am play-acting that I am a confident, happy person. The obsessional behaviour is still as strong as ever – for example, opening tins at the base to avoid any dust on top, folding tea towels with the pattern on the outside, jam pot lids with the printing and paper tags lined up with the label, toilet seats down after use, coat hangers facing the same way on the rail. These don't cause me a problem so I don't feel the need to change them.
>
> During the years since I finished therapy, I have joined day and evening college and have taken various courses including bricklaying, plumbing, welding, furniture restoration and French polishing. As these courses are normally taken by men, it would not have been possible for me to even consider taking them in the past. I feel totally comfortable doing them now. I feel more able to cope and get on with my life. I can even smile these days and mean it. **Eileen**

Pam

Pam was sexually and physically abused by her father and sexually abused by another family member. Her first husband was an older man, who also physically abused her. Pam has now achieved the professional qualifications she needed to pursue the career of her choice.

> I was married throughout my therapy but I have since divorced. I am now a career mum totally independent financially. I've struggled to get my career on track as a single parent but I've achieved it. I have qualified as a counsellor and also as a further education teacher/trainer/lecturer. I have been fortunate enough to work with survivors and with schizophrenic and PTSD clients. All of this work has enriched my life greatly. I have achieved more than I thought was possible when I was surviving my abuse and recovering. I am continually moving my goal-posts in order to meet a new challenge. I have recently started writing my own book about my life, my experiences, and post-therapy changes.
>
> I have learnt that I love my son immensely and that he is the most important thing in my life. I didn't believe in myself as a

mother, now I am a mother first. I'm not infallible, I'm human. I do my best and this is acceptable. This is the commitment I made to my son when I made the decision to have a child. I'm proud of the fact that I can combine a career, motherhood and run a home on my own. I've now got a wonderfully supportive relationship with my parents. I am a strong person and, I think, self-aware. I've become a professional independent woman. I know what I'm capable of. I know my limitations. I'm much more assertive and confident although this does wane at times. I've moved on from the dependent, unconfident, emotionally unstable person I once was, whose thoughts revolved around abuse. I'm now more confident, emotionally stable and satisfied. I feel fantastic. **Pam**

Ingrid, Kate, Fiona, Jane, Eileen and Pam all describe how they feel better about themselves, are more confident and act more assertively. Relationships of all kinds are better for them. Since therapy, they have all felt strong enough and free enough to pursue qualifications, careers, skills training or interests for themselves. Like Ingrid, they have all rebuilt their lives and have become truer to themselves.

Ingrid, Kate, Fiona, Jane, Eileen and Pam also reflect on what helped them in therapy and what has helped them since.

What helped

Being with others who had been through the same problems as me is what helped me the most. I remember listening to another survivor talking about her feelings and thinking 'that is what I feel!', and feeling relief at not being an outsider any more. Although I had talked to many health professionals, in my attempts to receive help before I finally found the Wakefield survivors' group, I never before had the feeling that I was truly understood or that I could share my feelings and thoughts.

Since therapy, I have learnt to see myself as a valuable person with the same rights as anybody else and because I express this in the way I behave this is also how I am treated by others. I have learnt to speak about my feelings, my thoughts and worries to those close to me. I have become confident and able to trust people. Having trust in people and not being disappointed reinforces the ability to trust. **Ingrid**

Most important for my recovery was the one-to-one counselling and group therapy I experienced at the Wakefield Psychology Service and the genuine support I received from Charles Fortte (who then worked for the Gracewell Foundation). Without his help, I don't think I would have ever told my mother. He also gave me an insight into offenders, which proved very valuable to me and to others as well. Healing is a continuing process. I feel that throughout my life I have been fortunate enough to meet many people and experience many different situations which have helped me to heal. I have also been helped by books and articles, attending training courses, work colleagues, friends and some family members. **Kate**

Being able to talk and explore the abuse and how it affected me, without being judged, was a great help. Being supported and respected by my therapist and the survivors' group members and being able to look at alternative ways of behaving was also very helpful. I now work as a counsellor and, in my profession, it is important to continue my journey of self-awareness and growth. **Fiona**

The healing initially involved being given time and space; being made to feel valued and worth helping; feeling I had something to offer as support for others; and recognizing and accepting support when I needed it. Being given the time and space to talk about my feelings and emotions allowed me to release feelings which I had held in for years. I was then able to put them aside and explore what I felt about a lot of other issues. The healing has continued and I know now when I need space, and I have friends who can give and receive support. **Jane**

The counselling was a godsend having spent 50 years denying that the abuse had happened to me as it was too painful to admit (even to myself) that the physical, mental and sexual abuse was reality. The group therapy and hearing other people's stories made me realize that I had lived a very lonely life believing that I was the only person in the world who had been abused. **Eileen**

The support of other group members really helped me. The relationships that were forged in therapy have continued to date. I feel lucky that these people are friends, close friends whom I can be open and honest with. We talk about all sorts. We still support each other through crises. We socialize together and have a laugh together. The relationships I now have with these people are as close as friends can be.

Every time I hit a crisis, my eating disorder emerges as something I can control while everything else seems out of my control. The healing process comes into play every time I encounter a crisis. I sit back and analyse, assess its impact, release the feelings, identify the options and put these into action. Once the crisis is overcome or dealt with, my eating disorder goes away again. It's almost a friend. I can deal with crises now because I learned to take control and to focus on the things that are important. Group therapy enabled me to analyse my life and take time out to re-evaluate what is meaningful. **Pam**

All the survivors emphasize the importance for healing of receiving support from others whether in individual counselling, from other survivors or from family and friends. This helped them to stop feeling worthless and alone. Feeling valued, understood and sharing their feelings without being judged also helped them overcome their problems. Being able to give and receive support continues to help them deal with the difficulties that are part of everyday life.

Does the abuse play any part in the lives of these survivors now?

Survivors often ask if they can ever truly put the abuse behind them. Eileen describes how she used to feel that her past was always with her, and Ingrid felt haunted by constant reminders of her abuse. How much are they affected by the abuse now?

The abuse is no longer at the forefront of my thoughts and it is very rare that I think about it at all. So much has happened in my life and I have changed so much that it almost seems like a totally different life I once led. I used to walk down the street, see someone wearing glasses and think 'my abuser wears glasses' or heard a certain phrase spoken and thought of him. Almost everything reminded me of my abuser and the abuse I suffered. Thoughts used to come uninvited and were almost constant reminders of a past I so much wanted to forget. The problems I had as a result of the abuse overshadowed every aspect of my life but now they are gone. When I met my abuser again, 5 years ago, I felt no fear and no inferiority. My fragile body image used to crumble when he was close but this time I felt no different, it was as if he had not been there. I am free. **Ingrid**

My own childhood abuse has no negative effect on my current life. The large number of problems I endured in my childhood gives me experience that helps me in my current work with clients. My past feelings and defences give me great insight which I use constructively in my work with counselling clients. **Fiona**

As a parent, I am concerned about child protection issues. I feel that many children are given inappropriate freedom without any experience of how to cope with it. I find it difficult to reconcile what my daughter's friends are allowed to do with what I feel is appropriate. This makes it harder to maintain firm boundaries with my daughter under such pressure from her friends. **Jane**

Until the therapy I always felt that the abuse was within, without and around my life continually every day. Now the abuse is in the past. Even though I will never forget the abusers and their actions, it is now behind me and I can get on with my life. The feeling of being trapped in my own body with a nightmare past no longer haunts me. I am extremely protective with my three grandchildren (girls). We play act what they would do and how they should react if they were approached by strangers, and discuss the differences between good touching and bad touching. **Eileen**

Working through the issues and difficulties arising from my own abuse allowed me to turn my negative childhood into something positive. I'm a better person because I know how it feels to be trapped, abused, used, beaten, betrayed, unloved. My own understanding of abuse has enabled me to pursue a worthwhile career – I now teach professionals on issues of child abuse and adult survivors. I don't think about the abuse at all unless I'm training other people about the subject. I am a parent who wants my child to feel loved and appreciated. I want to give him the best I possibly can. Most of all I want him to have happy memories of his childhood and I want to be there for him. There was a time when I could never imagine getting out of bed on a morning and the abuse not being there but it's happened. It's not there, it's no longer my waking thought. I don't think about the abuse any more. I enjoy life. I thought there could not be life after abuse but there is. **Pam**

Ingrid, Kate, Fiona, Jane, Eileen and Pam now feel free from the burden of their pasts. They have all begun to use their awareness about abuse in constructive ways. Jane, Eileen and Kate have described using their experiences to increase awareness of child abuse and child protection. Ingrid has since worked with victims of violence who have become perpetrators of violence. Pam and Fiona have found their own past experiences help them in their chosen careers.

Breaking free from your past and overcoming your problems is an ongoing process. Growth, healing and developing self-awareness continue throughout life. Ingrid, Kate, Fiona, Jane, Eileen and Pam have all continued to develop and grow. They continue to use the skills they have learnt and now see their abusers as 'in the past' and not part of their current lives. They have all made many positive changes and moved forward in their lives, and they know that for all of them, and all of us, the journey continues.

Appendix 1
Keeping safe, how to breathe properly and how to manage panic attacks

One of the most disturbing consequences of being sexually abused is feeling powerless and out of control. Most survivors feel anxious, and they often experience panic attacks, which makes them feel out of control and can be extremely frightening. Learning how to breathe properly, and knowing how to manage panic attacks, is the quickest and most effective way of getting in control of your emotions. If you have panic attacks or are overwhelmed by your own emotions, it is important that you keep yourself safe by reading this appendix, and practise breathing properly, before you work through this book.

When we are afraid, the natural reaction is to breathe very fast or to gasp more air (hyperventilation) to prepare ourselves for action (running away or fighting). Overbreathing like this can become a habit, so that people breathe too fast, or sigh a lot, even when they are not afraid.

How to breathe properly

The aim is for you to feel more in control by learning to breathe properly, so that the oxygen and carbon dioxide levels in your bloodstream become balanced. You need to learn to breathe from your diaphragm and to breathe slowly and calmly.

Speed of breathing

Use the second hand on a clock, or a stopwatch (you probably have one on your phone), as a timer. Try to breathe *as you normally do* for 1 minute (use a second timer), and count how many breaths (in and out is one breath) you take in 1 minute. **This should be between about 10 and 14 breaths per minute** while you are sitting around. (Obviously, it will be a lot more if you have recently exercised or run up the stairs, or are very worked up.)

If your breathing rate is higher than about 17 breaths per minute, you are probably hyperventilating. (Hyperventilating, or overbreathing, is just breathing more oxygen in than you need at the time.)

You should aim to breathe 10 to 14 breaths per minute. If you can make each breath (in and out) lasts for 5 seconds, you will be breathing at 12 breaths per minute.

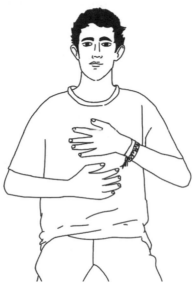

Figure 1 Breathing properly

- Put one hand on your chest and the other underneath lower down, over your diaphragm (see Figure 1).
- As you breathe in and out, notice which hand rises first. If it is your top hand, you are breathing to your chest and you are breathing too shallowly. Try to breathe more deeply so you can feel the bottom hand rising first. Your top hand should hardly move at all.
- When you breathe in, imagine you are filling up your lungs like a balloon, from the bottom up.
- Breathe in and out through your nose, if you can. Breathe in slowly and calmly. You do not need to put any effort into breathing out, just *slowly* let the air out of your lungs.

Practise breathing properly

- First make sure you can see the second hand on a clock or you have a second timer (for example, on your phone) with you.
- **Then breathe down to your diaphragm, as above, and try to make each breath (in and out) last for 5 seconds. Do this for at least 3 minutes.**
- When you first do this, you may feel a bit dizzy or light-headed afterwards. You are not used to breathing properly! This should settle down as you practise more – do not practise this while you are driving or using machinery. Continue to practise until you no longer feel light-headed afterwards.
- Many of you will feel calmer straight away.

Start with each breath lasting 5 seconds and try to gradually increase it to 6 or 7 seconds per breath if you can. You now have an easy way of calming yourself down!

Breathing correctly (as above) for 3 minutes will help correct any imbalance in your blood chemistry and get your oxygen and carbon dioxide levels back to normal.

Do this 3-minute breathing whenever you want to calm down or before you do anything (for example, go into a meeting, make a phone call, ask someone for a date, enter a shop) that makes you nervous.

Retrain your brain so you always breathe properly

If you have developed bad habits of overbreathing and have been chronically hyperventilating for a period of time, you need to retrain your brain.

- Breathe correctly (as above) for 10 minutes and *focus your attention* on your breathing (so don't do this while watching TV, drifting off to sleep and so on).
- Do this as many times a day as you can manage (at least 4 times). Log when you do it.
- Practise this regularly, for a month or so, until it becomes your natural way of breathing.
- You should then be breathing correctly in your day-to-day life – this should reduce your symptoms and help you feel calmer and more in control.

It will always be helpful to breathe this way, even if you *are* watching TV or doing your ironing, but to retrain your brain to always breathe properly, you need to pay attention to your breathing for 10 minutes as described above.

Panic attacks

What are panic attacks?

> I had to go to the hospital to see a doctor. I got a taxi there and sat in the waiting room. The clock seemed to be ticking really loud and everything seemed very noisy. I was called into the doctor's office. He was talking to me but I just couldn't hear what he was saying. I starting sweating and felt very hot. My hands were trembling and I couldn't stop swallowing. My chest felt tight and I felt the room was coming in on me. I just had to get out. **Polly**

We all feel panicky at times if we get a shock, or think we have lost our wallet, or a car swerves towards us. Panic attacks are an extreme form of anxiety or fear that comes on very suddenly and unexpectedly, and are very frightening. They are usually triggered by thoughts or memories, although we may not be aware of the trigger. The brain has an alarm system (in the amygdala, part of the limbic system) that goes off to warn us when we are in danger. Triggers related to past sexual abuse can set off the alarm even when you are not in any current real danger.

Panic attacks consist of:

- a very strong feeling of dread, or impending doom, or terror;
- a set of very powerful physical symptoms;
- a strong urge to run away.

People often react to these symptoms by thinking they are going to have a heart attack or die, or by thinking that something terrible is wrong with them. These thoughts make people even more frightened and so increase the physical symptoms and the tension. This in turn leads to more negative thoughts and causes the panic to build up and up.

People often think they cannot breathe and so they gasp for air, but this makes it worse because they have actually been breathing too much. They may also have hot or cold flushes and feel that their surroundings seem unreal, which can be very scary.

Many people who have panic attacks start to do things they *think* will prevent them from having an attack. For example:

- they always look down when walking along the street in case they get dizzy and have a panic attack;
- if they feel the symptoms coming on, they sit down and try not to move at all to prevent a heart attack or whatever they fear is going to happen;
- they gulp air because they think they cannot breathe.

These actions do **not** prevent a panic attack – the attack is caused by frightening thoughts and by overbreathing. In fact, acting like this will often make the fear worse. Test it out and see what happens by doing the opposite of these. For example:

- walk down the street looking around calmly and breathing slowly;
- walk around instead of sitting down;
- hold your breath, and then breathe very slowly instead of gulping air.

If you frequently experienced fear as a child, the alarm system in your brain may still be switched on so you are on alert for signs of danger all the time. This can result in you having panic attacks in the night as well as during the day. Although this is disorienting, you can cope with them in the same way as with daytime panics.

Taking control of panic attacks

I have to be strict with myself and know that even when I panic now it doesn't mean it's the end of the world. I try to stay where I am, breathe slowly and concentrate on telling myself, 'I can do it, I am certain to succeed'. I find this helps. **Polly**

Panic attacks are intense waves of anxiety. The most important thing to do is to control your breathing.

The steps listed below will help prevent panic attacks.

- Learn to control your anxiety – the more anxious you feel, the more likely you are to have a panic attack.
- Try not to perform avoidance behaviours, like looking down or gulping air, as these will usually make it worse.

- The most important thing is to make sure you are breathing properly; learning to breathe properly may eliminate or reduce panic attacks.
- Anxious and panicky feelings often trigger overbreathing; this sets you off on the path to having a panic attack. If you notice what is happening at this stage and start breathing slowly and calmly, you may be able to prevent a panic attack coming on.

If you start to have a panic attack, you will need to deal with the three parts of anxiety.

- **Physical symptoms: hold your breath if you can and then breathe out _really_ slowly.** Then continue to breathe as slowly and smoothly (not deeply) as you can until the symptoms die down. Try to relax your body. It is difficult to do something that _feels_ wrong (for example, holding your breath), but remember that one of the effects of overbreathing is that you _feel_ like you need more air. You don't. So try not to gasp for more air – this will only make the panic worse. Try to relax.
- **Behaviour:** stay where you are. Do not escape.
- **Control your thinking: think realistic thoughts,** such as:
  - 'I've had panic attacks before and they felt dreadful but nothing terrible happened.'
  - 'I know how to breathe properly now and I can control them.'
  - 'It's only a panic attack, it will soon pass.'
  - Don't focus on your physical symptoms – distract yourself by thinking of something else; for example, do a shopping list or mental arithmetic in your head.

If you do have a panic attack, remember that the symptoms peak within 10 minutes and usually only last between 5 and 10 minutes.

When you have a panic attack you may also experience a feeling of dread as if something awful is going to happen. In fact, the panic attack itself is the awful thing – nothing worse is going to happen. **A panic attack feels terrible but it is _not_ dangerous.** Fighting panic attacks can increase the fear; so just try to let the panic attack wash over you, don't fight it. Afterwards, take care of yourself; sit and relax and tell yourself it's over now and you are fine.

You *can* learn to control your breathing and your panic attacks, instead of feeling that they control your life, where you can go and what you can do.

Summary

Why not type the three main points below into the notes app on your smartphone or write them on a piece of card so you have them with you and can look at them whenever you feel a panic attack coming on?

If you feel a panic attack coming on, take the following steps.

- **Hold your breath and then breathe out *really* slowly.** Then continue to breathe as slowly and smoothly (not deeply) as you can until the symptoms die down.
- **Stay where you are.** Do not escape or run away from where you are (unless you are in real danger).
- **Think, 'It's only a panic attack, it will soon pass.'**

Appendix 2
Survivors speak out

This appendix contains the background stories of six of the survivors who contributed to this book. *Do not feel you have to read these stories.* They are included because some readers may want to know more about the histories of the survivors who have added quotes and examples to *Breaking Free*. The descriptions of the sexual abuse and its effects on the survivors are powerful and at times distressing, but their stories also contain the hope that they can already see a better future ahead.

Jane, Eileen, Anita, Graham and Pam speak out about the sexual abuse they suffered and how it has affected them, both as children and as adults. Each survivor's story is different, but many of the emotions and distress they experienced, and the consequences of the abuse on their lives, are similar.

You may feel upset for the person whose story you are reading, but the stories might also trigger feelings about your own abuse. Use these stories to reflect on your own experiences and feelings. If you can, find a friend to whom you can talk about how you are feeling. Read the appendix slowly and stop whenever you want to. Leave the stories and come back to them later *if you wish.*

Jane's story

I am in the bathroom staring at the light. I am lying on the floor next to the scales. I don't remember what my daddy said to me beforehand but I remember as he lay down on top of me. I wanted to push him away but he held my wrists to the floor on either side of my head. I remember his clothing rubbing against my naked skin. The contact hurt, the pressure hurt as he rubbed himself up and down over me. I remember his brown Crimplene tie flapping around my face. Afterwards he stood me in the bath water. He told me not to tell, that my mother would not understand, it was our secret. The threats came later.

That was the first time my stepfather sexually abused me. I was 7 years old. My parents split up when I was 4. My natural father had always been a distant figure, and then for 3 years I had very little contact with any men. When my mother remarried we became a proper family. My little sister and I had a daddy.

As the family became older my stepfather became more threatening and domineering. As I became older I felt that I was treading a tightrope between my two lives. I wanted to be liked and loved as me but what if people knew what I was really like, what I allowed to happen, what I was involved in? My stepfather was very popular, he used to collect pensions for the old, prescriptions for the sick, move coal for people and clear snow. So I thought it must be me that was really bad. I must be responsible. Who would believe otherwise? My stepfather used to reward me with money sometimes, more money than my mother could spare, so I felt even more guilty. I felt that if my mother found out, her marriage would break up. It would be as if she was being punished, not me, whose fault it really was.

Sometimes I would screw up all my courage and refuse him, but whatever tactics I employed he would outmanoeuvre me. He would appear to go along with me and then he would begin to be really nasty to the family. He would reduce my mother's housekeeping. He'd threaten to throw us all out of the house. He would go to the pub straight from work and be late home for meals. He would fluctuate between totally ignoring one of us and picking on us for minor things and blowing them up out of all proportion. He had total control over the TV and would change the channel 5 minutes before the end of a programme we were all watching. 'My name is on the rent book' was a popular phrase of his that would cause a fair amount of distress. He would then come back to me and ask again. This would continue until I gave in. I felt guilty for giving in to him and I felt guilty for causing all the misery to my family.

When I began to menstruate, I wanted to beg my mother not to tell him. I felt ashamed again, not in control of my body, but I didn't feel I had the right to ask her not to tell him. I wondered if this would change anything, but I guess since penetration wasn't involved nothing did change. I still used to have nightmares about becoming pregnant through clothing. Once I developed breasts (a word I didn't like as he used to tell me I had beautiful breasts) I only had to strip to my waist. He would change into nylon trousers and then push his nicotine stained tongue into my mouth and ears, and play with my nipples with his hard cracked fingers. I would be on the floor and as I silently cried the tears would collect in my ears. I could never work out why the sight of tears didn't put him off. I would clench my fists on the floor and grit my teeth against his tongue and try to imagine myself out of my body. I lived in constant dread – I knew what would happen whenever I was left alone with my stepfather. Being ill and off school was not much fun at our house.

Keeping this big secret made me feel I was different. I had to pretend that I was normal and the same as everyone else. I kept very much to myself, not daring to risk close friendships or to draw attention to myself in any way. I deliberately didn't take an active role in the classroom at school. I had friends at school but no best friend, no one to come home to tea. The more I pretended, the more guilt I felt over the deception and the more certain I became that people liked the 'pretend me' not the real me. The friends that I did have were mainly boys because they were happy to play outside rather than inside and they weren't interested in being 'gossipy'. I found them less socially demanding. This became a problem with my stepfather when he began to see them as a threat. I was about 14 at the time.

I have always been alone. I don't think I ever considered telling. I knew of no one who could cope with sharing this awful secret. Now I know that it wasn't my secret and I no longer feel isolated. Having met other survivors, I feel sad for what they have been through but it has helped me realize that being abused wasn't my fault. I don't have to be ashamed. I know now I am not alone, that the feelings that I had were not abnormal, and that I am not mad. Now I am free and I am in control of my life. I know who I am. I am full of hope for the future.

Postscript: In Chapter 17, 'The journey continues', Jane writes about what happened to her in the 7 years after she wrote her story.

Eileen's story

I think that my uncle must have sexually abused me from the age of 2 or 3 years old. I was told that I began to be a 'naughty child' about this age. I was continually disruptive from then onwards, which resulted in an application for early entry to school. I thought that if I did something really naughty someone might find out that Uncle was putting his hand down my panties and hurting me with his fingers. I played 'dare games' with my friends in the hope I would get hurt and would be taken to hospital and away from my uncle. My father was fighting the war and mother was still suffering from the death of my younger sister and didn't notice anything beyond my attention-seeking behaviour.

I started school on my fourth birthday. This was a year earlier than the usual age of acceptance in those days. Being sent to school early was a form of rejection to me and I resented being there. As soon as the teacher turned her back I ran away and arrived home before my mother by a different route. This was a daily routine for almost 3 years. The resentment built up in me even stronger as I was punished regularly. We lived one and a half miles away from school and my mother spent most of her day walking back and forth between home and school determined to get me used to it. I eventually did.

My mother and I visited my grandparents almost daily and I was regularly sent to deliver messages and to do errands for Uncle, who lived in the same street. My earliest memories are of knocking on Uncle's door. The door would open and I would be quickly pulled into the house. He would lock the door and push me against the wall beside the window and put his hands down my panties and touch me. He told me that if I told anyone what was happening I would be punished for what *I* had done wrong.

The feelings of guilt and fear increased in me. I felt very confused, helpless, dirty and disgusted. There was no one to talk to. I was very much alone and very lonely, I was desperately unhappy and cried silently for help but no one could hear me. There was constant pain and soreness in my genitals but no one noticed that either.

By the time I was 8 years old, he was partially penetrating my body with his penis. Although he did not climax at this time, he gained great pleasure from the abuse. At the age of 10 years I was suffering from gross anxiety and displaying more behaviour problems than ever. I had nightmares of his overweight stocky body, his thick spectacles and his aggressive manner in his excitement. His heavy breathing, and his sweaty hands as he held me down, repulsed me and I would wake up in the night, crying, afraid and shaking with fear. I began to have frequent bouts of vaginal pain on passing urine. I was unaware at the time that I was suffering from cystitis and that this was connected to the abuse.

By the time I was 11, the feelings of guilt and unhappiness were very prominent. I cried every night and lived in constant fear of the next attack. My personal hygiene became an obsession in order to cleanse my mind and body of the dirty feelings from the abuse which was forced upon me. I hated him for abusing me and gaining pleasure from it and causing me pain and misery. My vagina was constantly sore and the thought of his sperm seeping from my body following intercourse nauseated me. He obviously never stopped to think how I felt and only appeared to be concerned for his own selfish needs.

My school work suffered despite the struggle to learn. The abuse was always prominent in my thoughts and learning came second. I was encouraged by the school teacher to take the 11 plus examination. She said I had the ability but didn't apply it. I failed the exam miserably, possibly due to lack of knowledge, but mainly through lack of concentration. I constantly hoped that the teacher would guess the reason for my misery and poor school work. I was too young to realize that no one has a crystal ball in their head to read unspoken words and thoughts. I thought no one would want to help me, even if they could, as I was dirty, disgusting and unworthy of help. I was not even fit to be a human being because of the disgraceful things I did.

My abuse continued until one day at the age of 14 years he attempted to attack me as though it was his lawful right. He tried to pull me to the floor and started to grope his hand up my skirt. I began to struggle and fight, hitting him anywhere my fist would reach while avoiding his hands in resistance. He was very shocked at my reaction at first but soon recovered when I hit him on the face with one hand and at the same time pulled his hand away from tearing at my underwear. It was a hard struggle as he was a very strong man but miraculously I managed to get away from him. When I reached home, I burst into a flood of tears and, very briefly, told my father what had happened. He went to see my uncle. I never discovered what action my father took to resolve the situation but the abuse never occurred again. My parents obviously thought it was a 'one-off' incident. I was never asked and I didn't tell them otherwise. Possibly the reason they didn't ask me was that the abuser was a family member so it was kept quiet and covered up.

I carried the secret for 50 years as even in my adult life there was no one I could trust with my story. In the past years, the press has publicized stories of rape and abuse and the females have often been accused of provocation and of being the guilty party. On the strength of that I felt no one would believe me either. I had pushed the experiences of the abuse to the back of my mind and pretended it had not happened – or so I thought. That is, until the nightmares and flashbacks pushed it forward again. Whenever child abuse was publicized I always felt very sympathetic towards the abused and extremely angry at the abuser. It never occurred to me that I understood because it had happened to me. It would have been too painful to remember my childhood experiences and associate them with others who were suffering the same. I felt unworthy, dirty, disgusted, ashamed and unfit to be a human being. I felt depersonalized, detached and I had lost my personal identity. I became a victim of life.

Wrestling throughout my life with the emotional misery and torment of abuse has been very difficult but with determination and group therapy I have overcome the major difficulties in the emotional side of my life. The abuse has changed my personality and I have often wondered what or who I would have been without the traumatic experiences. I have been burdened by the misery of my emotions all my life up to the present time. I often think of the 'other me' and what it would be like to have had not only a happy contented childhood but also a peaceful and happy transit into adult life. Now I have been to a survivors' group and have told my story, maybe one day I will find the real me.

Postscript: in Chapter 17, 'The journey continues', Eileen writes about what happened to her in the 7 years after she wrote her story.

Anita's story

As I look back on my life and recall events leading up to my abuse, I have no happy memories at all. I'm sure there must have been some good times, but I really can't remember any. I had never felt loved and secure as a child. My father was for ever drunk and became very violent and abusive towards my mother. I was terrified of him. My mother was always tired and overworked and I can't remember ever seeing her smile. Neither of them ever gave me love or affection and I was desperate for a little love. I tried so hard to make them love me but I always got everything wrong. I was a shy, clumsy child and I was constantly put down and ridiculed at home and at school. As I grew older I became more and more shy and insecure. I had no friends and was desperately lonely.

Eventually my father left home and moved in with a girlfriend. At first he came to see us, but gradually his visits got less and less. My elder sister moved out to live with him and that was the last I saw of both of them. My mum by this time was working every hour God sends and I never saw her either. As I was now the eldest girl at 10 years old, I came home from school to an empty house, did all the housework and made a meal for my elder brother and younger sister.

Around the same time, I became very ill and was diagnosed diabetic. I spent 2 months in the hospital with no desire to get better at all. The only visitor I had in all that time was my mum and she found it really difficult to visit as she had to work. Because of this I felt very guilty. My mum had had a terrible life and now as it was just picking up I had to go and get ill and become an even greater burden than I was already.

While I was in the hospital my mother remarried and when I came home my stepfather made a terrible fuss of me. I felt so special, I had never had attention like this before and I loved it. In fact I made a point of showing off to my brother and sister. 'I'm his favourite', I'd say, 'He really loves me.' I threw myself at him. Every time he sat down I'd jump on his knee and throw my arms round him. He'd kiss and cuddle me and I felt so special. I immediately began to call him Daddy and was sure at last I did have a real daddy who really loved me. I soon began to realize that I didn't get cuddled so often when other people were around, but I put this down to him not wanting to make my brother and sister jealous. He began taking me for long rides in his car. He'd park in a lonely spot and then start to kiss me, but somehow the kisses weren't the same. They were sloppy and wet and I didn't like it. I daren't tell him though. He also started touching me all over my body. This made me feel uncomfortable as I really didn't understand it. It was a really funny feeling and I wished he wouldn't do it. Each time we went out he did this more and more. He also started breathing funny and I began to feel quite frightened.

My mum now was working most nights and he started telling me to stop up after the others went to bed. He told me he loved me, but I'd not to tell anybody, because no one would understand and I'd get into trouble. We'd keep these special times secret just between us because he loved me so much. 'And you do understand, Anita, it's because I love you so much that I do these things to you. Don't be frightened. I won't hurt you. You'll like it, I promise. I do love you.' But he did hurt me. It was horrible. He did terrible things to me and I was so frightened. He talked to me all the time telling me how wonderful everything was. 'It's good, isn't it, Anita? You like this, don't you? I told you you would, didn't I?' I was so scared I couldn't move. My body was stiff and tears were rolling down my cheeks. Yet still he seemed to be in a fantasy world believing I was really enjoying it.

He was so perverted and I feel sick at the thought of the things he did to me. As he became excited he began to slaver and dribble all over me and he'd grunt just like a pig. I tried so hard to cry out, I opened my mouth but nothing happened. I had now become quite ill and withdrawn. All the teachers put this down to my being diabetic. I didn't bother at all about my diabetes and made myself ill on purpose. On several occasions, I became so ill I was taken into hospital for investigations and re-stabilization and this was the only relief I ever got.

When I was 14 I had become such a freak at school I was a constant source of fun for the other kids. One day a couple of girls were making fun of me, referring to the fact I had never had a boyfriend and trying to embarrass me by asking me all sorts of silly questions about sex. Had I ever tried this or had that done to me? I became so fed up with it I broke down in tears and told them all to leave me alone because in actual fact I had had more experience than all of them and knew more than they'd ever know. One girl, though, persisted and wanted to know what I was talking about, so I told her. She was shocked and then insisted on dragging me off to our school counsellor.

I couldn't really tell the school counsellor anything, only that my stepfather had done things to me, which is all I ever said to anybody. He then told my mother. I was terrified of facing her, I felt as if I'd wrecked her life once again. Her first words to me were 'Why didn't you tell me? Why did you tell someone else?' This seemed to have really hurt her and I felt guiltier than ever. She promised me it wouldn't happen again and that was an end to it. It wasn't mentioned again. It did stop for a couple of weeks and then one day he came in to tell me how sorry he was. He began to cry and he put his arm round me, as he did so he began all over again. I later told my mother he had started doing things again and she said she'd make him stop. By this time, he seemed to have realized he could get away with anything and so now he didn't even wait for my mum to be out of the house. I never knew when he was going to appear next. I'd be certain he was out of the house so I'd risk running a bath and he seemingly appeared from nowhere.

My life was a nightmare. I decided the only answer to my problems was to end it all so I overdosed on my insulin and put myself in a coma. Of course I was saved, and sent to a child psychologist who told me all my problems were due to being called 'matchstick legs' as an infant. After this episode, I was quite desperate and took it upon myself one day to try out a pub. I found, with a little make-up and the right clothes, I looked quite attractive and easily got served. After this I found a way of numbing myself. I couldn't make the problem go away but at least I could make it bearable. I stopped going to school. I'd just disappear into the park with a bottle of vodka. The teachers never even seemed to notice. I started going out every night. I'd just walk into a pub and I'd always get drinks bought. I was 15 by this time and I'd just stopped caring.

I started getting invited to parties and the first time I went along to one I stayed out all night and when I got home he was waiting for me. He began to hit me. I thought he would never stop. He told me I'd worried my mother to death and how dare I do this. After that first time it was much easier. I told my mum I was going out and I didn't know if I'd be home and she seemed to accept this. I went out almost every night. I was always drunk and I slept around. I just didn't care. I smoked dope and took LSD, anything so I didn't have to feel.

Then one day the lad I spent the night with seemed to have become besotted with me and asked me to marry him. I was now 16 so I said 'Yes'. My mum agreed and that was that. A month later we were married. Soon afterwards I was rushed into the hospital with acute liver damage and was told I must treat alcohol as poison. I didn't take another drink for 3 years. Instead I became obsessed with having a baby and eventually after losing a couple I had a baby. This was the unconditional natural love I'd been waiting for all my life and it was all I wanted.

Our marriage was a joke. There was nothing between us, we each led separate lives, and I wouldn't have sex unless I really couldn't get out of it. I made excuse after excuse. Luckily the first time we did have sex, after our daughter was born, I fell pregnant again and so didn't have to bother until after the birth of our second child. After our son was born I had a lot of illnesses and used this as an excuse. I eventually had to have a big operation. When I got over this my husband became very impatient. He came home drunk one night and raped me. From this our third child was born and immediately afterwards my husband walked out and left us.

After this I became obsessed with dieting, and after a short period of anorexia I became bulimic [bingeing on food and vomiting] and this took over my life. It's the only way I have of coping with life, as deep down I really detest myself. I am desperately lonely and unhappy and I just can't wait for life to hurry up and finish. I've had a couple of disastrous relationships since the break-up of my marriage. I just can't seem to make them work. I hate sex and men and find it difficult to make friends generally with anybody. I keep trying hard to make my life work. I adore my children and I don't think I give them what they deserve, but I keep on trying and maybe one day I'll get it right.

It seems everything I try I fail at and the harder I try the bigger mess I make. I moved house and tried to make a new start shortly after the break-up of my marriage. The first time I gave in and accepted a little practical help from a man, I ended up being held prisoner in my own home for 3 days, being repeatedly raped and abused. I then got into a relationship with a man so manipulative and possessive it was like reliving my childhood all over again. After so many horrific experiences I wonder if maybe it's been me that's caused it all along. My own daughter was molested at 4 years old by a man at Butlin's holiday camp. I wonder if all men are abusers. Maybe they are normal and I am the one with a problem.

I have recently found a faith in God which has kept me going and helped me believe in myself more. I am now gaining confidence gradually and hopefully beginning a whole new life.

Postscript: Anita bravely tackled the problems resulting from her upbringing and the sexual abuse she suffered, and developed a successful career as a teacher.

Graham's story

My story is an account of the physical, mental and sexual abuse which I was subjected to from at least 5 years old. There are some memories from when I was even younger but they are vague and I can't make proper sense of them. Apparently, my aunt looked after me for the first year until my mother took me back – probably for the child benefit. I have always known that my mother didn't like me but it's hard to think she hadn't wanted me from birth. It would probably have been better if she had opted for an abortion rather than subject me to the life I have had.

For as long as I can remember my mother has always tried to hurt and embarrass me in front of friends or whoever else might be around. She always called me 'little bastard'. When I was little I drew on my face with a pen and she scrubbed my face until it was bleeding. Once she tried to kill me. She tried to drown me in the bath, holding my head under the water. I think it was because I got up with a soiled nappy. I can still see that face from under the water. She was slapping me and showing her fist as though she was going to thump me in the face. My head was in the water with my eyes wide open and I could see the anger in her face. I tried to breathe but my mouth and nose filled with water. I can remember struggling and then I was on the bathroom floor, coughing. She dragged me downstairs, pulled me across her knee and smacked me and told me not to do that again.

I was usually sent to bed at 7 o'clock and I cried myself to sleep. I never knew if I would wake up in my own bed or hers. She would go to bed around 11 o'clock and about half an hour later I would hear her pathetic voice calling me. I would pretend to be asleep, hoping she would stop. She never did stop. She would get louder and louder until I could detect her voice getting angry. I knew if I didn't answer her she would come marching into my room and literally drag me from my bed into hers. If she saw I had wet my bed she would smack me. It got to a point that I answered her straight away and got into her bed so I wouldn't be smacked for wetting the bed until the next morning. When I got into her bed she cuddled me and I didn't like this because I knew what was coming next. She would slowly rub her grubby hands all over my body. She would squeeze me closer to her and I would try to turn my head away from the smell of tobacco and beer. She would rub baby lotion between my legs and bottom. She would gradually get more aggressive, touching my genitals and squeezing them in her cupped hand. She would move her other hand under me and push her fingers into my bottom. It hurt me but I knew I had to try not to cry or she would get angry and smack me. After this she would move to the bottom edge of the bed and position herself rather like a woman having a baby. I can't get myself to say what happened next. I cannot cope even thinking about this, let alone living with it. It is fucking disgusting to me to live my life knowing she made me have sex and oral sex with her. It is so degrading and I try to forget, it hurts so much because she is my mother.

Her boyfriend used to come and stay for days on end. If I didn't do something they wanted me to do she would make me sleep naked in a larder all night and tell me Jack Frost or Dickie Dark was waiting for me. One night when she went out with her friends he stayed in to look after me. As soon as he was alone he sat me on his knee and put his hand under my bottom. He ended up with one of his fingers in my bottom. He put some sort of lubrication on his penis and had full anal sex and I screamed. It made me soil the bed and he slapped me for that and for crying because he hurt me. Up until then I had never experienced such pain. He gave me some money and told me this is our secret.

I am disgusted that I was often taken into their bed and told to do things to both of them. The things a decent parent wouldn't think of. I didn't know that having sex with her or with him was wrong because I'd never known anything else but I never understood why it used to hurt so much. It carried on right until she died and I am sure that if she was still alive it would still be going on now. I wished someone would help me and stop them hurting me. I tried to do what they told me to do because sometimes they were nice to me if I did it properly.

She used to let him take me to his house on Friday nights and he would take me back home on Sunday nights. She used to do some kind of preparation for when he came. She would pull my pants down and put me over her knee. She would put two suppositories in my bottom and tell me to sit on a potty. After a while she stopped using suppositories and would lay me on a table in the bathroom. She fixed a tube to the tap and put the other end up my bottom. She would turn the tap on and my abdomen used to swell up and it hurt like hell. She wasn't careful with me and she often made me bleed from my bottom which frightened me. She didn't care and made me wear a nappy, even to school, to stop the blood showing through my pants. It didn't stop either of them from having sex with me and penetrating me.

I didn't like going to his house. There were always other children there and one of the worst parts was being stripped naked and left with the other children in a toy room. There was also loads of adults. Some of them were nice but the others didn't even talk. I had to do some things to them like oral sex. Sometimes they would spank me, others pushed things into my bottom even though they knew it hurt me. There were a few who just wanted to treat me as their baby. My mother knew I was being taken to his house and used as a child prostitute with men, women and other children.

When I was about 9 years old I ran away. After 2 days my mother phoned the police who brought me home from the railway station where I'd been sleeping. I wish I'd told the police why I'd run away but I was frightened of what they would do to me and I knew it was all my fault and no one would believe me. When the police had gone my mother and her boyfriend made me strip naked then beat me all over my body with a belt until my body was covered with lash marks. From then on, I did everything they told me to do, no matter how dirty I thought it was.

My mother had many suicide attempts and I was always having to phone for an ambulance. She eventually killed herself when I was 15 years old. The last time I saw her boyfriend was when I was 17. I was on my way home after a night out in Leeds. He and three of his friends trapped me in a public toilet and decided to rape me, with two girls chanting and encouraging them on. They threw me around, thumped me and kicked me and I couldn't do anything but beg them to stop. He used the same phrase he always used: 'Are you going to be nice to me, we've got a lot to catch up on.' He started to undo his trousers and the other three dragged me up and literally tore my trousers and underpants off me. The two slags started to join in chanting 'fuck him, fuck him.' I will never forget that as long as I live. They anally raped me and made me perform oral sex. They left me bleeding and naked on the floor and told me they would find me if I reported it to the police. I locked myself in my bedsit for three weeks and was eventually sectioned and kept sedated in a psychiatric hospital for a year.

I don't know what it is like to have a mother. A mother who would show me affection and occasionally put her arms around me to make me feel safe and cared for. I hate myself and I have tried to get this out of me. I have washed, scrubbed and torn my skin to get the abusers off me. I take laxatives to get it all away from me but it won't go away. I feel ashamed and unclean and never feel as if my body or the house is clean enough. I have tried to kill myself many times but I won't do that now because I have my children to look after. At times the abuse seems to come flooding back to me. Even though my mother is dead, I still can't go into the bathroom without hearing her calling my name and I feel her pushing me. As well as these hallucinations, I have nightmares, flashbacks and panic attacks. The abuse has left me unable to show affection to my wife and children. I hate the torment I've put my wife and children through, shouting at them and shutting everyone and everything out of my life. I spent days on end secluded in my own room, I was punishing myself through a sea of bad memories.

A couple of years ago, I got into a very depressed state. I was going through a bad crisis in my life and I was getting no help or support from anywhere. My wife searched for help for me and found all the help was aimed at women. It made me feel that it is OK to rape a man and use a boy as a child prostitute. I eventually got a referral to clinical psychology. I dreaded seeing the psychologist and needed a lot of pushes from my wife but it wasn't as bad as I thought it would be. I felt a lot of relief. I have since been receiving weekly therapy sessions. It makes me feel better knowing that just talking to someone I trust frees me of some of the bad thoughts I had about myself. I feel a lot better in myself and, although I'm not at the end of my therapy yet, I am coping and can get on with life a lot better.

Postscript: with Graham's consent, we went to the police with all the information that Graham could remember about where the paedophile gang met to abuse all the young children, and with Graham's description of his mother's boyfriend who had organized the network of abusers. Unfortunately, due to the passage of time, there was not enough information for the police to track down the gang of abusers.

Pam's story

My mum and dad had to get married as I was an unexpected early arrival. All through my childhood I felt this was the reason they both treated me so badly. They never bought me clothes, shoes, school uniforms, and so on. They made me babysit my brother and two sisters and I had to do the housework, washing and ironing. I was a stand-in housewife in more ways than one.

One Saturday in August when I was 12 years old, my mum went shopping and as usual my father was left to look after us all. I went upstairs to wrap my mum's birthday present up. I couldn't manage so my dad came upstairs into my brother's bedroom, supposedly to help. As I was walking out of the door my dad grabbed me, pulled me on to the bed and ripped my shirt out of my skirt. I began to shout and scream and kick. Nobody came to help me.

He started fondling my body and sucking my breasts and then he pulled my pants down. I was still shouting and screaming and kicking. My brother came upstairs demanding, 'What's going on?' My dad threatened him with a beating, so my brother went back downstairs, none the wiser.

My dad kept trying to shut me up. He said I would enjoy it. After he had finished, he walked off leaving me crying into the pillow. He came back fully dressed shouting, 'Hurry up and get dressed before your mother gets back.' I walked into the bathroom. My father came in and pulled my bra back down and then left me.

For years my dad had made sexual comments to me, and tried to put me on the pill as soon as my periods began, but this was the first time he'd raped me. It went on for another 2 years. I had nightmares and daymares all the time. I became withdrawn, defiant and snappy. I felt as if my whole body was crawling. I felt so dirty and used. The same sort of thing had happened to me before, but with a different, older, member of the family. This left me wondering if I was different from everybody else. I was all alone. Fears of becoming pregnant constantly ran through my mind. I mentioned the rape to the NSPCC officer who was visiting our family at the time. He wasn't interested. My mother commented on my change of behaviour, so I told her. She said I was a liar and should have been drowned at birth. Nobody was willing to help, so I ran away and took an overdose, but it didn't work and I ended up back home.

At 17 years old I met and fell in love with my first husband who was 12 years my senior. I left home to live with him and we eventually got married, but he couldn't accept what had happened to me and also decided he didn't want any children. He turned out to be just like my father, he beat me regularly and so I left him and filed for divorce.

After my divorce my faith in men disappeared completely and the nightmares continued. Then 18 months later I met my second husband who guessed there was something wrong between me and my father, so I told him the story. He was the first person whom I had told and who had understood. Six months later I was pregnant and we had a son. One year later we married. Then I started suffering from depression and agoraphobia. I thought this was a build-up of trying to cope with a baby, work full time and falling out with my parents. After seeing my GP, I realized my problems were to do with the sexual abuse. She referred me to a psychiatrist, who wasn't much help as he was a man, but he referred me to a clinical psychologist who ran a group for women who had been abused as children.

During the group emotions ran high. I relived all the horrible episodes again, often beating my husband in my sleep, shouting and screaming at my father in my nightmares. I became very depressed. After about 10 weeks of the group I confronted my mother and father, by locking them in my house and telling them how much I hated them and why. At last my mother believed me. As soon as they had gone home I felt so much better for getting it off my chest, now the healing process could begin.

I am now in control of my emotions. I don't have nightmares any more and my marriage is even better for having gone through this trauma. I don't think I could have done it without the love, understanding and thoughtfulness of my husband whose love and devotion spurred me to get treatment in the first place.

I have now forgiven my father, although I will never forget. He knows this, my mum knows this and now we get on OK. We understand each other, and keep our distance. My life has meaning for the first time and I can honestly say, *there is life after abuse.*

Postscript: in Chapter 17, 'The journey continues', Pam writes about what happened to her in the 7 years after she wrote her story.

Sources of help

Note that if there is not a terrestrial address given in the contact details for an organization included in this section, it is because the organization wishes you to write via a form that can be found on its website.

The organizations are grouped under the following headings:

- In an emergency/helping children and young people at risk
- Telephone helplines/websites
- Therapy, counselling and support
- Sources of useful information

In an emergency/helping children and young people at risk

Stop it Now!
Bordesley Hall
The Holloway
Alvechurch
Birmingham B48 7QA
Tel.: 0808 1000 900 (confidential helpline)
Website: www.stopitnow.org.uk

If you are abusing children and young people, or have urges to abuse children and young people, then contact Stop it Now! immediately, on the confidential helpline or via the confidential email service (at: help@stopitnow.org.uk – your email address will not be displayed to preserve confidentiality; do not include your name in the email).

Alternatively, phone the NSPCC (see below), discuss this with your GP or contact the local authority or the police – but do talk to someone.

If you have any concerns about a child or young person who may be at risk, or about someone you know or suspect is a child abuser, it is important that you act straight away and get support and help from the appropriate specialist agencies. If you have suspicions, but no proof, it is still OK to contact the agencies below. You can contact them anonymously if you need to.

The police
If the child is in immediate danger, or in any other emergency, you can call the police on 999. If you want to contact the police when it's *not* an emergency, you can call 101 and ask to be put through to the specialist child protection investigation team.

The local authority
Local authorities are responsible for child welfare; you can contact the children's social care team if you are worried about the safety of any child. The team will have a 24-hour emergency number. This may be available on your local authority's website or on the website of your local Safeguarding Children Board. Alternatively, you can visit the following website and enter your postcode to find the telephone number of your local authority: www.gov.uk/report-child-abuse

NSPCC
Weston House
42 Curtain Road
London EC2A 3NH
Tel.: 0808 800 5000 (24-hour helpline for adults); 0800 1111 (Childline, for children and young people)
Website: www.nspcc.org.uk

The NSPCC has statutory powers. You can telephone the helpline for advice, without giving your name if necessary. You can find out more about the systems and laws concerning child protection in the UK at: www.nspcc.org.uk/preventing-abuse/child-protection-system

Samaritans
Freepost RSRB-KKBY-CYJK
PO Box 9090
Stirling FK8 2SA
Tel.: 116 123
Website: www.samaritans.org

Samaritans has a helpline that you can call to talk about anything that is worrying you. You don't have to be suicidal to contact Samaritans.

Legal help

In an emergency, you might need legal advice – if a child is being taken away immediately for his or her protection, for example. Often, local solicitors who specialize in child abuse cases run an out-of-hours service. Visit Survivors in Transition's website for information on how to contact child abuse lawyers.

Survivors in Transition
Support Centre
84 Fore Street
Ipswich
Suffolk IP4 1LB
Tel.: 07765 052282
Website: www.survivorsintransition.co.uk

Telephone helplines and websites

The telephone numbers and websites of various national organizations are listed below. For local sources of help, contact the national office or look on the organization's website. These organizations offer someone to talk to, advice and sometimes face-to-face counselling.

Child Exploitation and Online Protection (CEOP)
Website: www.ceop.police.uk

CEOP is part of the police National Crime Agency and works to protect children from harm online and sexual exploitation. You can report to the CEOP any online activity relating to child sexual abuse or child exploitation that concerns you.

Childline
Tel.: 0800 1111 (for children and young people)
Website: www.childline.org.uk

National Association for People Abused in Childhood (NAPAC)
Tel.: 0808 801 0331
Website: https://napac.org.uk

NSPCC
Tel.: 0808 800 5000 (24-hour helpline for adults)
Website: www.nspcc.org.uk

Therapy, counselling and support

For more information about therapy and therapists, please read the sections 'Getting help' and 'Finding an accredited therapist' at the beginning of Chapter 15, 'Overcoming the problems'.

- Your GP can refer you to the NHS to see a clinical psychologist, other psychotherapist or IAPT (Improving Access to Psychological Therapy) services team.
- There may be voluntary agencies that provide therapy in your area at low cost or free of charge.
- You may have the funds to pay for a private therapist yourself.

The main professional bodies that register and accredit counsellors and psychotherapists (they all provide lists of accredited practitioners) include the following:

- British Association for Behavioural and Cognitive Psychotherapies (BABCP) is the lead organization for CBT in the UK (www.babcp.com)
- British Association for Counselling and Psychotherapy (BACP) is one of the UK's largest professional bodies for counselling and psychotherapy (www.bacp.co.uk)
- British Psychological Society (BPS) provides a register of chartered psychologists (www.bps.org.uk)
- Health and Care Professions Council (HCPC) is a UK-wide health regulator, responsible for the statutory regulation of 15 different professions, including clinical psychology, and registration with the organization means that health professionals have met national standards for their professional training, performance and conduct (visit www.hpc-uk.org/audiences/registrants to check if a clinical psychologist is accredited)
- United Kingdom Council for Psychotherapy (UKCP) is the leading professional body for the education, training, accreditation and regulation of psychotherapists and psychotherapeutic counsellors and holds a national register of psychotherapists and psychotherapeutic counsellors, listing those practitioner members who meet exacting standards and training requirements, plus a specialist register for psychotherapists working with children and young people (www.psychotherapy.org.uk).

EMDR therapy

See Chapter 15 for a description of EMDR therapy.

EMDR UK and Ireland

Website: www.emdrassociation.org.uk

The professional association for EMDR clinicians, which can provide you with information about EMDR and help you to find an accredited EMDR therapist in the UK and Ireland.

EMDR Europe

Website: emdr-europe.org

Contact EMDR Europe to find an EMDR therapist in a range of European countries.

EMDR International Association

Website: www.emdria.org

The EMDR International Association covers the USA and other non-European countries.

Other agencies offering support and/or access to therapy

Children 1st

83 Whitehouse Loan
Edinburgh EH9 1AT
Tel.: 0131 446 2300
Website: www.children1st.org.uk

This is Scotland's national children's charity.

Citizens Advice

Tel.: 03444 111 444
Website: www.citizensadvice.org.uk

Citizens Advice provides free, confidential and independent advice to help people overcome their problems. The contact details for your local Citizens Advice can be found via the website.

DABS (Directory And Book Services)

Tel.: 07854 653118 (24-hour answerphone helpline)
Website: www.dabs.uk.com

DABS produces the National Resource Directory, which lists over 500 services, groups and organizations that help victims of abuse and sexual violence throughout the UK and Ireland, and accompanying resources and information sheets. It also provides Pathfinder – a signposting service that provides free support and information all over the UK and the Republic of Ireland to any individual or organization regarding issues to do with childhood abuse, incest and sexual violence.

Kidscape
2 Grosvenor Gardens
London SW1W 0DH
Tel.: 020 7730 3300
Website: www.kidscape.org.uk

This organization works to prevent bullying and protect children.

Mind
15–19 Broadway
Stratford
London E15 4BQ
Tel.: 0300 123 3393 (infoline)
Website: www.mind.org.uk

Mind provides a guide to mental health services, a telephone helpline and information leaflets.

Rape Crisis England and Wales
Tel: 0808 802 9999 (helpline)
Website: https://rapecrisis.org.uk

To find the nearest specialist Rape Crisis services, use the search facility at: https://rapecrisis.org.uk/centres.php

Relate
Tel.: 0300 100 1234
Website: www.relate.org.uk

Relate can help with relationship difficulties and sexual problems, including providing couple counselling. Visit the website to find a Relate service near you.

The Survivors Trust (TST)
Unit 2, Eastlands Court Business Centre
St Peter's Road
Rugby
Warwickshire CV21 3QP
Tel: 0808 801 0818 (helpline)
Website: www.thesurvivorstrust.org

TST is a UK-wide national umbrella agency of organizations that
offer support to those living with the consequences of rape, sexual
violence and childhood sexual abuse throughout the UK and
Ireland.

Victim Support
Tel.: 0808 168 9111 (helpline)
Website: www.victimsupport.org.uk

This organization coordinates nationwide Victim Support schemes.
Trained volunteers offer practical and emotional help to victims of
crime, including rape and sexual assault; they can also support you
through the process of prosecuting perpetrators.

Sources of useful information

DABS (Directory And Book Services)
Tel.: 07854 653118 (24-hour answerphone helpline)
Website: www.dabs.uk.com

Provides accredited specialist practitioner training, such as the
course 'Working creatively with survivors of childhood abuse and
sexual violence'.

From Report to Court: A handbook for adult survivors of sexual
violence
http://rightsofwomen.org.uk/wp-content/uploads/2016/11/
From-Report-to-Court-a-handbook-for-adult-survivors-of-sexual-
violence.pdf
    Published by Rights of Women (2014), this is a useful handbook
that takes you through all the steps from reporting abuse to going
through the court system.

Positive Outcomes for Dissociative Survivors (PODS)
3 Archers Court
Huntingdon PE29 6XG
Tel.: 0800 181 4420 (helpline)
Website: www.pods-online.org.uk

Provides help, support, information and training to help people recover from dissociative disorders and dissociation.

Stop it Now!
Bordesley Hall
The Holloway
Alvechurch
Birmingham B48 7QA
Tel.: 0808 1000 900 (confidential helpline)
Website: www.stopitnow.org.uk

Provides information on the prevention of sexual abuse.

Survivors in Transition
Support Centre
84 Fore Street
Ipswich
Suffolk IP4 1LB
Tel.: 07765 052282
Website: www.survivorsintransition.co.uk

A good resource for information about abuse, including sources of help for male and female survivors, people with learning disabilities, boarding school abuse survivors, ritual abuse survivors, Christian survivors, people with dissociative disorders and so on. It can also advise on how to contact child abuse lawyers and agencies for the prevention of abuse.

Further reading

Ainscough, Carolyn and Toon, Kay (2000) *Breaking Free Workbook: Practical help for survivors of child sexual abuse* (London: Sheldon Press)

This workbook develops the ideas in *Breaking Free* by setting out practical exercises for working step by step on the problems resulting from childhood sexual abuse. Intended as a self-help book, therapists have also found it helpful to work through the exercises with their clients.

Shapiro, F. (2012) *Getting Past Your Past: Take control of your life with self-help techniques from EMDR therapy* (New York: Rodale Books).

Shapiro, F. and Silk Forest, M. (2016) *EMDR: The breakthrough therapy for overcoming anxiety, stress, and trauma* (New York: Basic Books).

Parks, P. (1994) *Rescuing the 'Inner Child': Therapy for adults sexually abused as children* (London: Souvenir Press).

DABS (Directory And Book Services)
Tel.: 07854 653118 (24-hour answerphone helpline)
Website: www.dabs.uk.com

DABS produces helpful information sheets and a book list of over 450 titles in categories relating to sexual abuse and recovery.

Index